What doctors, health care professionals and researchers are discovering about tea tree oil...

"Tea tree oil encouraged more rapid healing without scarring, than conservative treatment."
  Dr. Henry Feinblatt, *Journal of the National Medical Association*.

"The results obtained in a variety of conditions when tea tree oil was first tried were most encouraging, a striking feature being that it dissolved pus and left the surfaces of infected wounds clean, so that its germicidal action became very effective without any apparent damage to the tissues. This was something new, as most effective germicides destroy tissue as well as bacteria."
  Dr. E. M. Humphrey, *Medical Journal of Australia*.

"It (tea tree oil) will help relieve the itch from the genital wart virus, from Candida, and from non-specific bacterial or fungal infection. It will relieve the symptoms as well as overcoming the infections..."
  Dr. S. Cabot, *The Use of Tea Tree Oil in Clinical Practice*

"Australian Melaleuca alternifolia oil (tea tree oil) in suitable dilutions was found to be highly effective in the treatment of trichomonal vaginitis, moniliasis, cervicitis and chronic endocervitis." Dr. E. Pena, *Journal of Obstetrics and Gynecology*

"Tea tree oil in the treatment of bacterial vaginitis may be a safe, non-toxic alternative to standard antibiotic treatment especially in pregnancy." Dr. Blackwell, British Medical Journal *Lancet*

"Tea tree oil offers a natural, less expensive, effective alternative to currently used drugs for the described conditions *(acne, herpes simplex, monilia of the throat and mouth, monila rashes, eczema, non-specific dermatitis, oral canker sores, pustules, fungus of the fingernails, and Tinea cruris, pedis, and barbae)* in this study. It is safe, easily accessible and its side-effects profile superior to most products currently prescribed for these medical problems."
  A. Shemesh and W. Mayo in San Juan Capistrano, California, *International Journal of Alternative and Complementary Medicine*

The
Tea Tree Oil
Bible

Your Essential Guide
for
Health, Beauty, Home, Plant & Pet Care Use

Dr. Elvis Ali, N.D.
Dr. George Grant, Ph.D.
Dr. Selim Nakla, M.D.
Don Patel
Ken Vegotsky

AGES Publications™
Los Angeles, California & Toronto, Ontario

THE LOVE LIVING & LIVE LOVING HEALTH SERIES™

Library of Congress Cataloging-in-Publication Data

Ali, Elvis A.
     The tea tree oil bible : how to use it for health, beauty, plant &
pet care / by Dr. Elvis Ali & Ken Vegotsky.
        p.   cm. — (The love living and live loving series)
     Includes bibliographical references and index.
     ISBN 1-886508-10-0
     1. Melaleuca alternifolia oil.   I. Vegotsky, Ken, 1951– .
II. Title. III. Series.
RM666.M357A45 1998
615'.32376—dc21   98-3881
                                    CIP

Cover Illustration by Joerg Kilian, KilDe – KILIAN DESIGN
http://www.kilde.com

Book Design by Inside Bestsellers Design Group™ (800) 595-1955

Quantity discounted orders available for groups. Please make enquiries to Bulk Sales Department Tel. 1 800 263-1991 or Fax 1 800 458-0025

Printing history 02 01 00 99 ** 7 6 5
Printed in Canada. Published simultaneously in U.S.A. and Canada.

Transactional Reporting Service
Authorization to photocopy items for internal or personal use, or the internal use of specific clients, is granted by Ken Vegotsky the copyright owner, provided that the appropriate fee is paid directly to Copyright Clearance Center, 222 Rosewood Drive, Danvers MA 01923 USA

Academic Permission Service
Prior to photocopying items for educational classroom use, please contact the Copyright Clearance Center, Customer Service, 222 Rosewood Drive, Danvers MA 01923, USA (508) 750-8400

We dedicate this book to you, the reader.

To those who are seeking gentle and safe natural alternatives for healing, health and well-being.

To those women and men who are using the psychological transformational path outlined in The Ultimate Power for study groups, to enhance and change their life.

You are making a difference, each and every day.

Mission Statement

We vow each and every day, to share with you the miracles we have found in this greatest of gifts called life. Our mission is not to change the world but fine tune it for our children, all children.

Elvis Ali, George Grant
Selim Nakla, Don Patel
& Ken Vegotsky

We acknowledge with thanks:

The medical, health care and numerous other professionals who made this book possible.

The supportive people from the Melaleuca consumer direct group who provided samples of their excellent tea tree products.

Raymond Aaron for his encouragement.

Aloe and the incredible design team at Inside BestSellers Design Group.

The fine folks at Thursday Plantation Laboratories for their help, encouragement and assistance, and for providing a copy of and permission to use the pure Tea Tree Oil Certificate of Analysis in this book. A special thank you to Robert Riedl whose technical advise and editorial comments helped make sure this book had the most current and up to date information about tea tree oil.

The alternative and traditional print, radio and TV media, who support our efforts to make this a better world.

We are forever thankful to these fine folks who started the ball rolling. Tony, Chris and Charlette of KSON, Deborah Ray and Tom Connolly of the Nationally Syndicated show *Here's To Your Health* , Jana & Ted Bart and Karlin Evins of the show *Beyond Reason* on the Bart Evins Broadcasting Co. Network, Greg Lanning and Dr. Joseph Michelli, of the *Wishing You Well Show* on the Business Radio Network, Kim Mason of *The Nightside Show* on 1010 AM, Willa and Bob McLean of *McLean & Company*, *Canada AM* and *Eye On Toronto*, *Concepts Magazine*, Tony Ricciuto of *The Niagara Falls Review*, Julia Woodford of *Common Ground & Vitality Magazines*, Susan Schwartz of *The Gazette*, Casey Korstanje of *The Spectator*, Tess Kalinowski of *The London Free Press*, Len Butcher & Dr. David Saul of *The Tribune*, Joanne Tedesco of *The Arizona Networking News*, Andre Escaravage of *The Journal of Alternative Therapies*, Tony Trupiano host *Your Health Alternatives* WPON 1460 AM, Joe Mazza & Sabastion the Wonderdog of *The Joe Mazza Show* on Talk America.

The support of Mark Victor Hansen, New York Times #1 co-author of the *Chicken Soup for the Soul series*, Brian Tracy author *Maximum Achievement*, Jerry Jenkins of *Small Press Magazine*, Barry Seltzer, Lawyer and author, *It Takes 2 Judges to Try a Cow and Other Strange Legal Twists*, Dr. J. Siegel, Psychologist, Cavett Robert, Chairman Emeritus of the *National Speakers Association*, Hennie Bekker, *Juno Award Nominee*, Dr. Michael Greenwood, M.B.,B. Chir., Dip. Acup., C.C.F.P., F.R.S.A., co-author *Paradox and Healing*, Dottie Walters, President of Walters Speakers Bureaus International and author *Speak & Grow Rich*.

Dave, Nancy and Ian Christie, Mark Field, Marilyn and Tom Ross, Jerry Jenkins, Barbara Cooper-Haas, Sam Seigel along with a host of others, too numerous to list.

My children, Stephanie and Alan, who brighten my life immeasurably. Mom for being there, you are special. Joni, Robbie, Amanda and Ryan for being the wonderful family they are. Louis Alaimo, the best paver anyone can have do a driveway, but more importantly a great friend, thanks for being there. Sevi for being a friend who is down to earth. Barry Seltzer for being a lawyer, whom I've come to know is a human being first. Sheila and Lee, for being authentic.

Mom's incredibly supportive friends: Margot & Colman Levy, Florence & Eli Abranson, Lil Rolbin, Natalie Rosenhek and Sara Shugar. Their souls shine brightly in all they say and do. – *Ken Vegotsky*

To my lovely wife, Khadija, and our children, Hassan, Azeeda and Kareem, who inspire and motivate me to teach everyone about naturopathic medicine. A special thanks to my sisters, Alima, Anna and Lily, for their support. Most important of all, my wonderful parents, Hakim and Hazrah, who have always blessed and assisted me throughout my medical schooling. My wonderful grandmother, Mymoon, who always taught us to respect and care about others. – *Elvis Ali*

Finally, the most important person of all at this time - *you!* The reader. Your efforts to make this a healthier, more environmentally safe world and become a better person by buying this book are the greatest acknowledgment of support we can get. Together we are making this a better world by using safer, natural healing ways – one person at a time.
– *George Grant, Selim Nakla and Don Patel*

...Keep on making a difference!

Preface

Tea tree oil is a great all purpose essential oil. The purpose of this book is to give you and your doctor or health care practitioner as much information as possible in a clear, simple and concise manner.

What got us interested in tea tree oil were the many successful personal health and hygiene usages we and others were using on a daily basis. The overwhelming amount of testimonials, indicated a little known, yet powerful healing agent was being overlooked by the public.

In many cases, people did not have enough information to minimize their efforts and maximize the benefits to themselves. When used properly, tea tree oil can help you save time, energy and money. In essence you can become your own manufacturer and save time, energy and expense by keeping a few key products in your home, to use as a base for tea tree oil mixtures, or by boosting the effectiveness of products you are are already using by adding a few drops of this powerful essential oil. Many commercially produced tea tree oil products are now being made for consumers.

This explosion of interest started us on a journey of exploration, where we discovered documented studies of the safe and effective uses for this miraculous essential oil. A summary of the research, resources and sources are supplied. This will help your health care professionals in their quest for better and safer ways of delivering your health care needs. This will help you help yourself.

As in all matters of health and well-being, it is your responsibility to find the answers that work best for you. Self-health care is your constitutional right, one which you can exercise on a daily basis.

Share this book with your family, doctor and other health care practitioners, so they become aware of the versatile, therapeutic and healing powers of tea tree oil—nature's first aid kit in a bottle!

Table of Contents

Abscesses, Aches and Pains–Muscular, Acne,
AIDS, Arthritis, Athlete's Foot, Bad Breath,
Balanitis, Barber's Rash, Bee Stings,
Blackheads, Blocked Nasal Passages, Boils,
Bronchitis, Bronchial Congestion, Bruises and
Bumps, Bunions, Burns and Sunburn, Bursitis,
Calluses, Canker Sores, Candida Albicans,
Carbuncles, Carpal Tunnel Syndrome,
Chapped Lips, Chickenpox, Chiggers,
Chilblains, Chronic Fatigue, Clavus, Colds,
Cold Sores, Congestion, Coral Cuts, Corns,
Coughs, Crabs, Cradle Cap, Cramps, Cuticles,
Cuts and Abrasions, Cracked Dry Skin,
Cystitis, Dandruff, Dental Plaque, Dermatitis,
Dhobi Itch, Diaper Rash, Diabetic Gangrene,
Earaches, Ear Infections, Ear Wax, Eczema,
Emphysema, Fever, Flu, Foot Odor, Fungal
Infections, Furuncle, Genital Herpes,
Genitourinary Infections, Gingivitis, Gout,
Head Cold, Head Lice, Hemorrhoids, Herpes
Simplex type 1, Herpes Simplex type 2, Hives,
Hepatitis, Immune System–to Strengthen,
Impetigo, Ingrown Nails, Ingrown Toenails,

Insect Bites, Itching, Leeches, Lice, Leg Ulcers, Leucorrhoea, Measles, Moniliasis, Mouth and Gum Infections, Mouth Ulcers, Muscular Aches and Pains, Nails—infected, Nasal Passages—Blocked, Nettle Rash, Nipples—sore, Ovarian Cysts, Paronychia, Pediculosis, Piles, Pimples, Plantar Warts, Poison Ivy, Poison Oak, Prickly Heat, Pruritis, Psoriasis, Respiratory Tract Infections, Rheumatism, Ringworm, Salpingitis, Scabies, Shaving Rash, Shingles, Sinusitis, Sinus Passages, Sore Nipples, Sore Throat, Splinters—infected, Sprains, Stiff Muscles, Stiff Neck, Styes, Sunburn, Surgery—uses in, Sweaty Feet, Thrush, Ticks, Tinea, Tooth Ache, Tonsillitis, Ulcers—Varicose and Tropical, Varicose Veins, Urethritis, Vaginal Infections, Vaginitis, Veruccae, Veruccae plantaris, Warts, Wasp Sting, Wounds, Zona

The
Tea Tree Oil
Bible

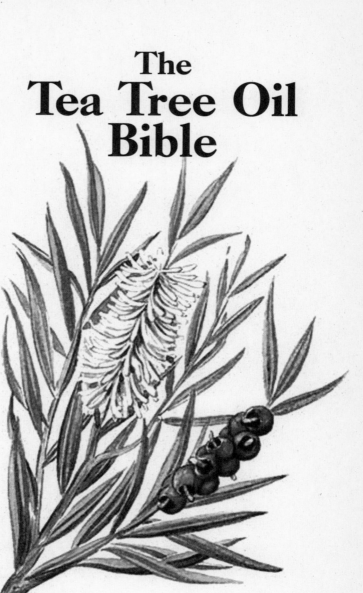

Melaleuca alternifolia

CHAPTER 1

What is Tea Tree Oil?

Tea tree oil is the essential oil from the leaves of the Australian Melaleuca alternifolia tree, a member of the botanical family Myrtaceae. There are over three hundred varieties of tea tree growing in the wilds of Australia. Many of them produce essential oils with healing properties. However, only one, Melaleuca alternifolia, has outstanding medicinal, beauty aid, personal hygiene, pet, plant and home care cleaning properties.

This tree grows in the Richmond River basin near Lismore, on the north coast of New South Wales as well as in the areas further south near Sydney and Newcastle. Yet, the botanical properties of their oils are sufficiently different that the tea tree grown in the north is preferred over those from the southern regions.

Why? Chemistry. A high terpinen-4-ol content combined with a low cineole content helps this variety have a safer and wider range of therapeutic uses. Terpinen-4-ol has a wide range of beneficial properties, with no side effects. Cineole's medicinal qualities are good for relief of colds. Recent scientific work indicates cineole is a relatively weak antimicrobial agent and is not irritating to the skin. Skin irritation may occur if the oil has a high para-cymene content. The

> *The way to health is to have an aromatic bath and a scented massage every day.*
>
> *Hippocrates*

northern variety of Melaleuca alternifolia is prized for its high terpinen-4-ol content and low cineole content.

Modern farming, planting, processing and quality assurance testing insures a superior product with a wide range of uses.

The latter part of the twentieth century has seen an explosion of interest in this miraculous plant. Modern cultivation and farming methods are now experimenting with producing this high quality tea tree plant in other areas. The growth of public awareness in alternative and natural healing products is causing the need for greater production of this essential oil.

Today, you will find Melaleuca alternifolia being grown in California and more farm lands being devoted to it in Australia.

Tea tree oil, also known a 'Ti-tree oil', from the Melaleuca alternifolia tree, is your first aid kit in a bottle. One you should never leave home without and never be without at home!

CHAPTER 2

A Brief History and Initial Studies

Archeological investigations indicate that the Australian Aboriginal people have lived on the continent over 40,000 years. Their existence depended on their peaceful coexistence with their environment and the plant and animal life that flourished there. Learning to live in harmony with their environment, they took what they needed from the land, waters and forests and no more. When injured or sick they found healing remedies in the strong medicinal properties of the continent's plant life.

In 1770 Captain Cook discovered Australia on a journey of exploration for the British. The Western World's first known collector of tea tree leave samples was Sir Joseph Banks who accompanied Captain Cook on his journey. He apparently was not aware of the healing properties of the plant. For many years only the Aborigines and a few settlers living in New South Wales were aware of the therapeutic value of the tea tree. It was not until the twentieth century that the scientific community began to take notice of Melaleuca alternifolia.

In 1922, a government chemist, Dr. Arthur Penfold, *FCS*, working as the curator and economic chemist for the Museum of Technology and Applied Sciences in Sydney, started a series of laboratory studies examining the antiseptic power of tea tree oil. He announced his results in 1925. According to the generally accepted standards of the time, tea tree oil exhibited bactericidal and antiseptic qualities 13 times stronger than carbolic acid. In addition to that, his research showed it was non-toxic and non-irritating.

In 1925 he announced his findings to the Royal Society of New South Wales. In 1929, Penfold and Morrison published their findings in the *Technological Museum Bulletin*.[1] The result was a burst of research in general medical practices and by the scientific community.

During the years following his initial research, his colleagues in the medical community started putting tea tree oil to the test. Initially it was tested as an antiseptic/bactericidal agent for numerous problems.

In 1930, the *Medical Journal of Australia* featured an article by E. M. Humphrey about tea tree oil, titled 'A New Australian Germicide.' He wrote:

> *The results obtained in a variety of conditions when it was first tried were most encouraging, a striking feature being that it dissolved pus and left the surfaces of infected wounds clean, so that its germicidal action became very effective without any apparent damage to the tissues. This was something new, as most effective germicides destroy tissue as well as bacteria.*

Other conditions that Humphrey indicated tea tree oil was good for included:

- Use as an antiseptic mouthwash in dentistry
- Infections of the naso-pharynx
- Powerful antibacterial deodorant properties
- Strong disinfecting properties on the typhoid bacilli indicating it was more than 60 times stronger than ordinary hand soap.

In the following years many applications were tested and studies made examining the therapeutic and numerous other claims about tea tree oil. Initially papers were published in *The Australian Journal of Dentistry*, *The Medical Journal of Australia*[2], *The Manufacturing Chemist*[3], *Soap and Sanitary Chemicals*[4], *Perfumes, Cosmetics and Soap*[5] and *The Australian Journal of Pharmacy*[6]. As tea tree oils reputation became better known, additional studies were reported in *The Journal of the*

National Medical Association of America and *The British Medical Journal*. In 1936 a severe life threatening case of diabetic gangrene was successfully treated and reported in *The Medical Journal of Australia*.

Worldwide interest increased and numerous reports from other countries indicated tea tree oil's power in treating mouth and throat infections, gynecological problems, parasitic and fungal skin conditions as well as its incredible antiseptic properties. Towards the end of the 1930's tea tree oil became known as a *miracle healer*.

How highly regarded was tea tree oil by the medical establishment and government of that era? At the outbreak of the Second World War it was standard issue in the Australian armed forces first-aid kits. Growers and processors were exempted from military service, to ensure adequate supplies of tea tree oil. Even ammunition plants used it in a 1 percent dilution in munition plant machine cutting oils to reduce skin infections to the hands, due to injuries caused by metal filings.

Unfortunately, tea tree oil's popularity waned with the advent of the synthetic pharmacological industries rise to power. The general public and medical establishment looked to man-made chemicals for the answer to their health care needs. The shift away from inexpensive natural remedies to highly profitable and patentable man-made drugs had begun.

CHAPTER 3

Additional Medical and Clinical Research Reports

The Second World War was the beginning of the era of synthetic germicides. Only in Australia did tea tree oil stay popular as a natural remedy.

It wasn't until the 1960's that awareness of the hazardous side-effects of many synthetic drugs, as well as their questionable costs and environmental implications, began to come under scrutiny by members of the medical research community.

Another issue contributing to the lack of interest, by pharmacologically based medicinal businesses, in natural alternatives, is the economic reality of the marketplace. Naturally occurring substances, in an unprocessed state, cannot be patented. This means that pharmaceutical monopolies, where the business can charge sufficiently high enough prices to recoup the costs for testing and research, could not be created. Today it is estimated to cost between 100 million to 300 million dollars to develop and complete the necessary testing for a new synthetic drug, before bringing it to the marketplace. Even then, that does not guarantee the company will ever recover its costs, let alone make a profit on its labors. The realities of business are ever present.

> *Naturally occurring substances, in an unprocessed state, cannot be patented.*

In America and Canada, this resulted in a lack of funding for medical and drug researchers into natural remedies. Even though research into alternative therapies continued around the world, particularly in the Far East, Europe and Australia, the findings were not being reported to the general public. The result of this is that America and Canada account for roughly 75% of the dollar value of world-wide pharmacological drug sales, yet represent only 5% of the worlds total population!

Even in Europe, the sales of pharmacological synthetic drugs, are relatively small in comparison. Yet the awakening of the 1960's started resulting in new research and reports about natural remedies.

Unfortunately, little media attention was paid to these findings, since money to publicize and advertise the findings was very limited. Both the public and media embraced sensationalism and quick fix mentalities.

In addition, American and Canadian government agencies and regulations were created to sustain and maintain the pharmacologically based businesses, which are highly profitable and excellent sources of tax revenues, jobs, and heavy financial supporters of traditional medical schools and associations.

Coincidentally, the 1960's saw the beginning of a resurgence of research into the numerous benefits of tea tree oil. Many studies are cited here, to give you an idea of the extensive research the tea tree essential oil, from the *Melaleuca alternifolia* tree, is garnering.

In the 1990's industry and consumer awareness of this essential oils powerful properties is fueling a growing world wide market. The Australian Tea Tree Industry Association, through private investors, raised 60 million dollars for a research and product development facility for tea tree oil. The research facility is being run in association with Southern Cross University in Lismore, Australia.

In 1996, an American multi-level marketing company, with over sixty products using tea tree oil, did $300 million of business and is expanding its consumer market share into Canada, Taiwan, Japan and elsewhere. Colgate-Palmolive tested a tea tree oil toothpaste, but could not secure sufficient supplies of tea tree oil to launch the product in other countries. The result was they discontinued making it.

Hospitals in Australia use tea tree oil to control mold and other pathogens in their environments.

In California, farmers are growing *Melaleuca alternifolia* trees, in an attempt to cash in on this fast growing and developing commercial market. Increased production, combined with industry and consumer awareness, indicates this is the beginning of a booming market for this renewable, biodegradable, therapeutic, non-staining, non-toxic and multi-purpose essential oil.

Hopefully, the economic potential for tea tree oil, will cause additional research to uncover all that this miraculous oil has to offer and other practical ways to effectively use it. The following is a sampling of some of the more current research, starting in the 1960's, up to the 1990's:

Source: *The Journal of the National Medical Association*, 1960

Paper: 'Cajeput - Type Oil for the Treatment of Furunculosis'

Content: Dr. Henry Feinblatt reported using pure tea tree oil, twice daily to treat 25 cases of boils (furunculosis), with success.

Results: In 8 days, 15 cases were completely cured, 6 boils were reduced in size by over half, 3 were greatly reduced, only 1 needed incision.

Conclusion: Tea tree oil 'encouraged more rapid healing without scarring than conservative treatment'.[7]

Source: *Journal of Obstetrics and Gynecology*, 1962

Content: Dr. E. Pena did a clinical study of 130 women with various types of vaginal infection - Candida albicans (thrush), cervicitis and trichomonal vaginitis. Used Melaleuca alternifolia, in a specially emulsified 40% solution of pure oil.

Results: Clinical cure rate of 100%

Conclusion: He wrote: *'Australian* Melaleuca Alternifolia *oil in suitable dilutions was found to be highly effective in the treatment of trichomonal vaginitis, moniliasis, cervicitis and chronic endocervitis... Daily vaginal douches with 0.4 per cent of the oil in one*

*quart of water proved safe and effective in treat-
ment of the vaginal infections under consideration.*[8]

Source: *Current Pediatry,* 1972
Content: Dr. M. Walker studied numerous foot problems -
athlete's foot, callouses, fungal infections and
under nail corns.
Results: Of the 60 patients treated with pure tea tree oil,
58 were cured. This was over a period of 3 weeks
to 6 years.
Conclusion: Excellent results occurred in 38 cases. Fair
effects in 20 cases.[9]

Source: *Planta Medica,* 1974
Researchers: D. Low, B.D. Rowal & W.Q.J. Griffin
Paper: 'Antibacterial Action of the Essential Oils of
Some Australian Myrtaceae' vol. 26:184, 1974
Conclusion: Tea tree essential oil is a superior bactericide.

Source: *Perfumer and Flavorist,* 1979
Paper: 'Bacteriostatic Activity of Some Australian
Essential Oils'.
Content: M.F Beyleir indicated very favorable results using
tea tree oil on the reduction of bacteria.[10]

Source: *Phytotherapy,*[11] 1985
Content: Professor P. Belaiche at the University of Paris,
Phytotherapy Department did a series of studies
with tea tree oil.
Study: Pure tea tree oil was used to treat a variety of
fungal infections (paronychia and nailbed infections) and skin condition disorders (acne and
impetigo).
Results: Generally positive.

Study: One involved 28 women, with the vaginal infection thrush (Candida albicans). For 30 days,
vaginal capsules infused with tea tree oil were

inserted every evening.

Results: Twenty-one women were completely healed. Seven women were clinically healed yet not biologically cured.

Study: A double-blind test was done with 26 women suffering from chronic cystitis. Half were given 24 mg of tea tree oil, in 8 mg doses, 3 times daily before each meal. The other half were given a placebo.

Results: Seven out of 13 from the first group were cured after 6 months. None of those on the placebo were cured.[11]

Source: The Associated Foodstuff Laboratories of Australia, 1983

Content: Skin sterilization studies, using tea tree essential oil, applied to unwashed hands.

Results: Hands washed in distilled water reduced from a count of 3,000 bacteria per 50 square centimeters to 2,000 per 50 square centimeter. Hands washed using tea tree essential oil had a bacteria count reduced from 3,000 per 50 square centimeters to 3 per 50 square centimeters. Tea tree oil effectively killed 99.9% of the bacteria upon contact.

Source: *Australian Journal of Pharmacy*, 1990

Paper: 'A comparative study of tea-tree oil versus benzoyl peroxide in the treatment of acne'

Content: Bassett, Pannowitz and Professor R. Barnetson of the University of Sydney and Dr. Phillip Altman, a specialist in pharmaceutical consultancy, conducted a study in the treatment of acne, involving 124 students, to evaluate the efficacy and skin tolerance of a 5% tea tree oil gel versus a widely used acne treatment with 5% benzoyl peroxide lotion.

Results: Tea tree oil took longer to take effect and was

equally successful. The essential oil had the added advantage of causing significantly fewer side effects.

Conclusion: Increased and better concentrations of tea tree oil may prove to be faster acting then the benzoyl peroxide lotion and not cause any ill-effects.[12]

Source: Conference proceedings on Modern Phytotherapy - the Clinical Significance of Tea Tree Oil and Other Essential Oils, from the December 1 & 2, 1990 conference at Macquarie University in Sydney, Australia

Conclusion: Dr. S. Cabot, in his presentation, *The Use of Tea Tree Oil in Clinical Practice* said, *"It (tea tree oil) will help relieve the itch from the genital wart virus, from Candida, and from non-specific bacterial or fungal infection. It will relieve the symptoms as well as overcoming the infections..."*

Source: *Lancet*, 1991
Content: Dr. Blackwell of the Department of Genitourinary Medicine in Wales reported on a patient who used 200 milligrams of tea tree oil in a vegetable base oil (vaginal pessary) instead of using metronidazole, the standard pharmaceutical drug to treat her vaginal infection.

Results: In six days the infection cleared up.

Conclusion: Dr. Blackwell concluded, *'tea tree oil in the treatment of bacterial vaginitis may be a safe, non-toxic alternative to standard antibiotic treatment especially in pregnancy'.*[13]

Source: *International Journal of Alternative and Complementary Medicine*, 1991
Content: A. Shemesh and W. Mayo in San Juan Capistrano, California conducted a more generalized study of the usefulness of tea tree oil in creams, as an oil and lozenges to treat the following conditions: acne, herpes simplex,

monilia of the throat and mouth, monila rashes, eczema, non-specific dermatitis, oral canker sores, pustules, fungus of the fingernails, and Tinea cruris, pedis, and barbae. The test group consisted of 2 children, 18 men and 30 women.

Results: Only one patient with eczema was resistant to the treatment. All others showed remarkable improvement or were cured.

Conclusion: A. Shemesh and W. Mayo wrote: *'Tea tree oil offers a natural, less expensive, effective alternative to currently used drugs for the described conditions in this study. It is safe, easily accessible and its side-effects profile superior to most products currently prescribed for these medical problems'.*[14]

Source: *Journal of Antimicrobial Chemotherapy,* 1995

Content: Carson, Cookson, Farrelly and Rilley reported on the 'Susceptibility of methicillin-resistant *Staphylococcus aureus* to the essential oil of Melaleuca alternifolia' in-vitro. The cultures of the bacteria were measured when dilutions of 0.2%-2.0% of tea tree oil were added. The bacteria were effectively inhibited at a tea tree dosage of 0.25% and killed at a 0.5% or greater dosage.

Conclusion: Tea tree oil may be an effective treatment to reduce transmission of methicillin resistant *Staphylococcus aureus.*[15]

Increasing evidence of the safety and multiple uses of tea tree oil to treat health related and other conditions are resulting in a worldwide expansion of production and distribution of this essential oil. It is now available in the U.S.A., Canada, Australia, New Zealand, United Kingdom, Finland, France, Italy, Israel, Malaysia, Korea, Singapore, Holland plus other countries.

Increased interest and studies are resulting in many new applications for this versatile essential oil. The December 1990 conference proceedings on Modern Phytotherapy - the Clinical

Significance of Tea Tree Oil and Other Essential Oils, at Macquarie University in Sydney, Australia reported on a wide range of studies about tea tree oil. R. Ryan, presented a paper on 'Oil of *Melaleuca alternifolia* Dissolved in Liquid Carbon Dioxide Propellant Used for the Control of Bacteria and Fungi in Air Conditioning Systems'[16]. The conclusion was positive. Commonwealth Industrial Gases has a treatment program for air conditioning ducts in large buildings. Their tea tree oil and carbon dioxide combination, called Bactigas™, is used to create a Healthizone™ in the buildings. The system uses the air conditioning system as a means of dispersing and distributing a controlled dose of tea tree oil at regular intervals. This inhibits the formation of bacteria, fungi and mold which thrive in the moist, warm, dark conduits which pipe the air through the buildings. The result is better quality breathable air, less molds on walls, less contamination of food processing areas, less respiratory infections and other benefits which occur when this system is in operation.

Additional information presented at the 1990 Macquarie University conference[21-35 incl.] indicates further lines of research and other uses for tea tree oil in these and other areas:

- Agricultural applications including pest control, delousing sheep, tick treatments, collar rot for orchard trees and the list continues to grow.

- Tests are underway indicating tea tree oil is an effective and non-toxic post harvest treatment for strawberries, mangoes and other fruit. Initial results are encouraging and hopefully one day the currently used, potentially poisonous treatments will no longer be necessary.

- Treating fungi in carpets and ridding houses of vermin such as cockroaches and fleas have gotten good results.

There are numerous grades of tea tree oil from the *Melaleuca alternifolia* tree and if the one you are using, is not working, it may not be of sufficient quality and strength or be an adulterated product. Try another brand.

If your skin is getting irritated, this usually indicates a lower quality of a tea tree oil with too high a percentage of para-cymene in it. Studies indicate adults can safely use tea tree oil effectively to deal with many conditions.

If you are concerned, call the supplier or check with your doctor or health care professional before testing out another brand of tea tree oil. When you meet with your health care provider, bring along the tea tree oil you used and another brand of tea tree oil. A simple test for adverse reactions is to apply a drop of the pure oil on your skin and wait an hour or two in their office waiting room.

Only pure, 100% unadulterated (no fillers) tea tree oil, from the Melaleuca alternifolia tree, is used to create the treatment recommendations in this book. Due to the highly concentrated nature of pure tea tree essential oil, it is measured by the drop.

Buyer beware. Read the label. If you are not sure of the product's quality, contact the manufacturer. Do not confuse price with value. A very small bottle of pure tea tree essential oil goes a long way and lasts years, when stored and used properly.

The list of proven applications using pure tea tree oil is extensive and growing in the industrial, commercial and consumer markets.

CHAPTER 4

Quality and Chemistry of Tea Tree Oil

An Essential Oil Primer

Currently, the most effective and therapeutic tea tree oil is the essential oil from the leaves of the '*Melaleuca alternifolia*' tree, grown in a 200 square kilometer region of New South Wales, Australia. Pure essential botanical oils are used in aromatherapy for their therapeutic healing properties. Aromatherapy uses the essential oils that are distilled from a whole plant or a specific part of the plant. It takes approximately 2,000 pounds of Melaleuca alternifolia leaves to get 20 pounds of distilled essential tea tree oil. That is the liquid equivalent of 11 quarts or 10.4 liters of tea tree oil.

The leaves are manually or mechanically harvested, after flowering, usually during the spring and early summer months, since this is when the best quality of oil is produced by the tree. This is a very labor intensive process. The Melaleuca alternifolia trees are very hardy and respond very well to the harvesting with renewed vigor and growth.

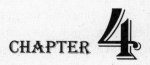

Tea tree oil is a truly unique essential oil due to the extensive diversity of benefits it offers!

The original bush method of steam distillation, had the leaves being placed in racks inside a steamer. The water was heated so steam passed through the leaves, bursting their oil sacks. This released the essential oil into a collection tank. The tea tree oil then floated to the top, since it does not mix with water, and was then filtered into containers. This method is giving way to a modern approach.

Today, many plantations generate the steam in a separate boiler. The steam then goes into a distillation pot and passes through the leaves. Using this method it only takes two to three hours to produce, condense and separate the oil. The discarded leaves are recycled as fertilizer for the fields. Each batch of oil is then tested for its chemical composition, thus insuring consistent standards of quality. Different chemical compositions have various uses. The highest standards are applied to tea tree oil being used for medicinal purposes.

An essential oil can contain as many as 200 organic chemicals, the combination determines the essential oil's properties. The Melaleuca alternifolia oil has close to 100 organic chemical components. For those requiring precise information about the chemical analysis of tea tree oil, refer to the article, 'The Composition of Australian Tea Tree Oil' by G. Sword and G.L. Hunter, *Journal of Agricultural Food Chemistry*, American Chemical Society, Volume 37, no. 5, 1989.

Different essential oils have a variety of beneficial effects on and in the body. They are very delicate and volatile. Improper processing, storage or exposure to sun, heat or air and they can easily lose their beneficial properties. With proper storage a small bottle will last years. A little really goes a long way.

The molecules of most botanical essential oils are smaller then the pores in human skin. This is why the body easily and rapidly absorbs the oils. These concentrated organic chemicals are absorbed by the bloodstream and distributed throughout the vascular (blood) system. The uniqueness of essential oils is that they appear to target specific systems in the body. This process offers numerous beneficial results. Tea tree oil is a truly unique essential oil due to the extensive diversity of benefits it offers!

Over the course of human development we grew in partnership with the world around us. Just as we use plant life to survive, they use us. For example, when we exhale we expel a waste product called carbon dioxide, which is what plants require to grow. In return plants get rid of their waste product called oxygen, which we require for our survival. Aromatherapy and the use of essential oils is part of a special and unique relationship plants and humans share. Modern methods of cultivation and processing have enabled us to create top quality therapeutic grades of essential oils.

When using essential oils to create aromatherapy massage oils, it is preferable to use organically produced, 100% pure botanical essential oils with the appropriate carrier base oils or products. Synthetic essential oils do not have the same or as broad a range of therapeutic properties as 100% pure botanical ones.

Though specific elements, such as the olfactory note (smell) may be able to be synthetically reproduced and duplicated, the synthetic essential oil rarely, if ever, duplicates the diversity of beneficial organic chemicals found in 100% pure botanical oils.

Read the labels to see if it is diluted in a carrier base or is 100% natural. For tea tree oil, the label should indicate it is from *Melaleuca alternifolia*, otherwise it can be from another variety of tea tree. If you are not sure, call the company and find out.

The purer and better balanced the concentration of medicinal chemicals in the oil, the better the likelihood it will have therapeutic properties you want. Smell does not necessarily indicate it is a 100% pure botanical oil.

If you are seeking therapeutic benefits from an essential oil, it is very important that you get the very best you can afford. In our opinion, that is unadulterated organically produced, 100% pure botanical essential oils. Buyer be savvy. Buyer beware. Read labels. Ask questions.

Excerpt from Stress Free Living: 222 Ways to Live Stress Free
Elvis Ali, George Grant & Ken Vegotsky, AGES Publications.
To order a copy please refer to the back of this book.

The Key Chemical Composition of Tea Tree Oil

There are over 300 varieties of tea tree plants. Some varieties of tea tree oil contain up to 200 chemical components. Only Melaleuca alternifolia has demonstrated the organic chemistry that provides such a powerful and wide ranging set of beneficial uses. Even among Melaleuca alternifolia trees, grown in the same region, there can be a large difference in the chemical composition of the oil.

There are close to 100 chemicals in the tea tree oil from the Melaleuca alternifolia tree. The key ingredients in this variety of tea tree essential oil are the terpinen-4-ol and cineole content. High levels of terpinen-4-ol are an indication of the oils ability to promote healing. A low cineole content is also important for therapeutic purposes. It is primarily the balance between these two chemicals which is used to determine the best grades of this oil.

In 1948 researchers took a random sampling from 49 trees growing in the north coast region of New South Wales, Australia. Their findings showed a significant difference ranging from 6% to 16% in their cineole content. High cineole content is not good for healing wounds and inflammations. Cineole does have beneficial medicinal qualities and helps relieve colds.

The Australian Tea Tree Industry Association mandates the terms for authentic certification of tea tree oil. Only oil produced by the Melaleuca alternifolia tree is acceptable.

In addition the Australian standard number AS 2782-1985 for Melaleuca Oil requires a terpinen-4-ol content greater than 30% and a cineole content less than 15%. This indicates how important it is for you to get your tea tree oil from a reputable supplier, with a quality brand. Avoid unsatisfactory blends and fraudulent concoctions which are passed off as genuine tea tree oil.

We say this after having bought numerous essential oil products which were misleading by their deceptive labeling. One major retailer promotes their aromatherapy products as being beneficial, focusing on the smell. Fortunately we asked the clerk about one of their products, did not get a satisfactory answer and called the companies' head office, only to discover the product was a blend with less than 10% by volume of the actual essential oil. On two counts it struck out, it was not a 100% pure botanical essential oil and it was highly diluted in a carrier base that was not appropriate for the therapeutic properties we were planning to use it for.

Government labeling laws may allow producers to say *100%*

Pure Essential Oil. Just like a label saying *100% Pure Concentrated Orange Juice* is okay, when you read the fine print you may discover it says water added. We cannot stress enough, that if you are looking to get a therapeutic benefit from the tea tree oil you purchase, make sure the supplier and source are both top notch quality!

Page 38 shows an example of the analysis of a batch of pure tea tree oil from a reputable supplier, Thursday Plantation.

Medicinal and other properties of tea tree oil

The tea tree oil from the Melaleuca Alternifolia tree has numerous properties making it very effective for a wide range of applications. In terms of therapeutic possibilities it is powerful against three main varieties of organisms - bacteria, fungi and viruses. Independent testing has shown its microbiological action against a large range of micro-organisms. The following is a list of infectious organisms tea tree oil has shown itself to be effective against.

Gram Positive bacteria:

Beta haemolytic streptococcus
Propionibacterium acnes
Streptococcus agalactiae
Staphyloccus aureus
Staphyloccus epidermidis
Streptococcus faecalis
Streptococcus pneumoniae
Streptococcus pyrogenes

Gram Negative bacteria:

Citrobacter spp.
Escherichia coli
Klebsiella pneumoniae
Legionella spp.
Proteus mirabilis
Pseudomonas aeruginosa
Shigella sonnei

Fungal organisms:

Aspergillus niger
Aspergillus flavus
Candida albicans
Microsporum canis
Microsporum gypseum
Thermoactinomycetes vulgaris
Trichophyton mentagrophytes
Trichophyton rubrum

Thursday Plantation

Health from Plants

**Thursday Plantation
Laboratories Limited**
ACN 002 833 141

Certificate of Analysis

Test Item	Results
Product:	Pure Tea Tree Oil
Batch/Identification Number:	#709034
Date Manufactured	Apr 1997

Test	Specification	Results
Description:	Colourless to pale yellow liquid.	Complies
Odour:	Myristic	Complies
Terpinen-4-ol:	≥ 35%	44.81%
1,8-Cineole:	< 6.0%	2.95%
α- Terpinene	5.0% - 13.0%	9.40%
γ- Terpinene	10.0 - 28.0%	21.24%
ρ- Cymene	0.5% - 12.0%	2.29%
α- Terpineol	1.5% - 8.0%	3.34%
α- Pinene	1.0% - 6.0%	2.16%
α- Terpinolene	1.5% - 5.0%	3.33%
d - Limonene	0.5% - 4.0%	0.79%
Expiry Date:	Apr 2002	
Storage Conditions:	Away from direct light. Below 30° C	

This product complies with Thursday Plantation Laboratories Ltd Specification Number : TPLS - 002.

This batch of product is released for sale.

Approved   *Wallis*
              Ceri Wallis.
              Quality Assurance Manager

Date   20/2/98

Pacific Highway Ballina NSW 2478 Australia
Telephone: (02) 6686 7273 Facsimile (02) 6686 7485 International Fax +61 2 6686 7485
www.thursdayplantation.com   email: teatree@om.com.au
The Original Tea Tree Plantation and the Finest Name in Tea Tree Products
OFFICES IN: • California USA • Virginia USA • Hampshire UK • Hong Kong • Malaysia • Sydney NSW Australia

Quality System

Quality
Endorsed
Company
ISO 9001 LIC1666
Standard Australia

Melaleuca consumer direct group sells tea tree oil based on the terpinen-4-ol and cineole content. Their guaranteed grades are T36-C7, T36-C5, T40-C5 & T40-C3. T40-C3 is a superior consumer guaranteed grade available in the U.S.A

In addition, tea tree oil offers therapeutic advantages that in conjunction with the above independently verified properties makes it even more beneficial as a medicinal. It stimulates the immune system, which means it empowers the body to better use its own natural wisdom to heal itself when threatened by these organisms.

The essential oil from the Melaleuca alternifolia tree is used in many products for one or a combination of these benefits that have been allegorically shared or demonstrated in clinical or laboratory environments: antifungal, anti-viral, immuno-stimulant, antiseptic/bactericidal, penetrating, solvent, expectorant, anti-inflammatory and analgesic. It does not stain and is generally considered non-toxic, yet care must be used with it or any essential oil, due to their highly concentrated levels.

Overview of Tea Tree Oil's Properties & Uses

Antifungal

Tea tree oil's antifungal properties make it very beneficial in the treatment of athlete's foot, ringworm and conditions caused by Candida albicans such as thrush.

Additional benefits include combating fungal diseases that affect animals, fish and plant life.

Antiseptic/Bactericidal

What this means is that it is an excellent first aid treatment for burns, cuts, infected splinters, insect bites, wounds of many types, including those that are dirty or contain pus. For general skin care it is an excellent antiseptic in the treatment of acne, blackheads, etcetera. Tea tree oil's general disinfectant properties make it a valuable tool against genitourinary tract infections such as cystitis and respiratory problems such as bronchitis and sinusitis.

Anti-viral

Currently there are no known effective synthetic drugs in wide use, that can inexpensively fight viral infections. Viruses are the cause of many epidemic illnesses. This is where tea tree oil offers a relatively safe, effective and inexpensive treatment, generally unknown to many traditional health care practitioners. Its powerful anti-viral properties makes it very useful against many common viral infectious diseases and problems. The following is a partial list: chicken pox, colds, cold sores, flu, measles, shingles and warts.

Immuno-stimulant

Tea tree oil is a valuable preventative remedy, helping the body use its own wisdom to fight off infection. Weakened states can be caused by antibiotics, drug use, illness, and stress in its many forms. These are five major sources of stress: chemical, environmental, emotional, mental and physical. What these conditions cause is a lowering of the body's natural resistance levels.

Further research is needed to explore tea tree oil's full potential for building up the immune system's strength before surgery. For use in people suffering from long standing or chronic conditions such as glandular fever, hepatitis and AIDS.

To discover numerous ways you can effectively deal with stress, see *Stress Free Living: 222 Ways to Live Stress Free* by Elvis Ali N.D., Dr. George Grant Ph.D. and Ken Vegotsky, AGES Publications. Ordering information is at the back of this book.

Additional properties of this amazing essential oil

Conditions effecting the skin, such as bruises, burns and cuts, benefit from tea tree oil's pain-killing (analgesic), anti-inflammatory and wound healing (cicatrizant) properties. Tea tree oil is seven times more soothing then aloe vera.

Problems such as lice, mosquitoes, scabies and other types of insect and parasite infestations are greatly benefited by tea tree oils insecticide and parasiticide properties.

Tea tree oils have a diaphoretic effect, which means it taps into the bodies natural preventative response against infection with its ability to promote sweating when the body needs to.

Tea tree oil displays balsamic and expectorant properties. These are very beneficial for chest and throat infections. In addition it is soothing and helps clear mucus from the respiratory tract.

Tea tree oil is aromatic.

It has penetrating properties, which make it excellent for use in industrial and household products.

Tea tree oil is a natural solvent which makes it very beneficial for biodegradable cleaning products in the home and workplace.

Bactericidal testing for antimicrobial effectiveness of tea tree oil may lead The Food and Drug Administration[17] (FDA) to list numerous therapeutic uses for tea tree oil for such conditions as hemorrhoids, ingrown toenails, Poison Ivy and jock itch.

CHAPTER 5

General Methods for Using
Tea Tree Essential Oil

Basically there are four ways to use tea tree essential oil; orally without swallowing, topically on the skin, internally for certain conditions and inhalation through the nose and mouth. Ingestion or swallowing, is currently not recommended, unless it is a commercially prepared tea. This section is an overview of various methods for using tea tree oil.

Tea tree oil is not miscible, it does not dissolve nor is it easily evenly dispersed in water, unless it is properly prepared beforehand. In general, oils and water do not blend well. To discover what we mean, put a few drops of pure tea tree oil in water, shake well, then let the container rest on a flat surface. Within ten minutes you will see oil droplets floating on the surface of the mixture. No matter how much you mix tea tree oil and water, the oil will not stay evenly distributed in the water when left to stand for a while.

The key to overcoming this problem, so the tea tree oil stays evenly dispersed in a solution, is to do an intermediary step by preparing a water-soluble tea tree oil concentrate. You may use the water soluble solutions the same way you use 100% full-strength tea tree oil, or you may dilute it with other materials, such as aloe vera gel, KY jelly, vitamin E ointment, herbal tea or water, depending on the use you are going to put it to.

Three Water-soluble Tea Tree Oil Mixtures

Always use a glass container or clear plastic one, with a good sealing top, for mixtures. Dark or amber colored glass containers are best for long term storage. Pure tea tree oil dissolves some plastics.

Measurements are rounded off and given in conventional and standard international metric units. In America standard international units are used by scientists and their students.

Only the United States and Burma do not use metric as their principal unit of measurement. Repeated attempts and Congressional legislation mandating the use of metric measurements exists, yet resistance to them has prevented the general use of metric.

Throughout the book both systems are referred to. This book is user friendly. All necessary calculations have been made for you and there will be no need for you to refer back to this information. The measurements given in the recommendations are as accurate as needed for the suggested use. Here are the conventional American liquid measurements and their standard international equivalents:

1 tsp	=	1/3 tbsp	=	1/6 oz	=	4.9 ml
3 tsp	=	1 tbsp	=	1/2 oz	=	14.8 ml
6 tsp	=	2 tbsp	=	1 oz	=	29.6 ml
1 oz	=	2 tbsp	=	0.0296 l	=	29.6 ml
1 c	=	16 tbsp	=	8 oz	=	236.6 ml
1 l	=	1.0567 qt	=	33.814 oz	=	4.2268 c
1 l	=	1000 ml	=	2.113 pt		
20 drops	=	1/30 oz	=	1 ml		

Pure Tea Tree Essential Oil
is measured in drops due to its high concentration.

tsp – teaspoon	tbsp – tablespoon	c – cup	pt – pint
oz – fluid ounce	qt – liquid quart	ml – milliliter	l – liter

Water-soluble Blend for External Use Only

Isopropyl Alcohol Base (rubbing alcohol base)

A small amount of isopropyl alcohol easily dissolves tea tree oil. The following are some of the conditions this isopropyl alcohol mixture is beneficial for: athlete's foot, burns, cuts and jock itch.

This mixture should never be swallowed, used orally or by inhalation. Keep away from eyes and other delicate or highly sensitive tissue. Isopropyl alcohol is toxic. Use it in lotions to treat external skin conditions only!

Equipment: Use a glass or clear plastic container with a good sealing top.

Formula: Blend 1 tbsp (1/2 oz, 15 ml) of isopropyl alcohol and 2 tbsp (1 oz, 30 ml) of 100% pure botanical tea tree oil. Shake vigorously. Let the bottle rest on a flat surface for a couple of minutes. If oil floats to the surface, add more alcohol and shake again, until oil is evenly dispersed in the mixture.

Be sure to clearly label the glass bottle you store this mixture in, with a warning and description of contents. The label should read *Water Soluble Tea Tree Oil in Isopropyl Alcohol base – EXTERNAL USE ONLY.*

Internal and External Use – Orally, Inhalation, Topical

Grain alcohol base mixture

The amount of grain alcohol it takes to dissolve the tea tree oil depends on how high a proof, percentage of alcohol to water content, is in the grain alcohol. A 150 proof grain alcohol is 75% alcohol and 25% water. A 100 proof grain alcohol is 50% alcohol and 50% water. And so on.

This mixture may be used with aloe vera gel, herbal tea, water or juice. It can be used as a body wash, foot treatment, mouthwash, vaginal douche, pet spray, plant spray and a host of other uses described in the following sections.

Equipment: Use a glass or clear plastic container with a good sealing top for this mixture.

Formula: In the container first add the grain alcohol according to the volume amounts below. Next put in the tea tree oil. Tightly seal the container and shake the mixture vigorously.

Test to see if the tea tree oil is evenly dispersed. Place the jar and mixture on a flat surface or counter top and let it stand for a couple of minutes. If a thin film or drops of the oil appear on the surface, add more alcohol and shake vigorously until the oil is fully dissolved. The mixture is okay and the tea tree oil is fully dispersed when the container looks uniformly cloudy.

Any distilled spirits may be used for this purpose, such as brandy, gin, rum, vodka or whatever. Most aromatherapists and herbalists prefer a neutral grain alcohol, such as vodka, since they are fragrance free.

If using a 192 proof alcohol, such as Everclear or a similar brand, start with 2 tbsp (1 oz, 30 ml) of high-proof grain alcohol and mix with the same amount of tea tree oil—2 tbsp (1 oz, 30 ml)—equal amount of alcohol to pure tea tree oil.

A 151-proof rum is the next best choice. Mix 3 tbsp (1 1/2 oz, 44 ml) of high-proof grain alcohol plus 2 tbsp (1 oz, 30 ml) of tea tree oil—3 parts alcohol to 2 parts pure tea tree oil.

When using an 80-proof alcohol, mix 6 tbsp (3 oz, 89 ml) of high-proof grain alcohol plus 2 tbsp (1 oz, 30 ml) of tea tree oil—6 parts alcohol to 2 parts tea tree oil.

Label the container *Water Soluble Concentrated Tea Tree Oil Mixture in a Grain Alcohol Base – Oral, Inhalation & Topical.*

Glycerin base mixture

Animal glycerin, made from cattle bones, is available in drug stores. Aromatherapists and herbalists prefer vegetable glycerin, which is usually available in herbal supply shops and health food stores.

In children's formula, alcohol based mixtures are not recommended, that is when you want to use glycerin. The sweet taste of glycerin makes it a popular solvent for making tinctures, adding a sweet taste to mouthwashes, a soft emollient touch to skin lotions such as after shaves, hand, foot and facial applications, etcetera.

This mixture may be used with aloe vera gel, herbal tea, juice or water. It is good for a body wash, foot treatment, mouthwash, vaginal douche, pet spray, plant spray and a host of other uses described in the following sections.

Equipment: Use a glass or clear plastic container with a good sealing top for this mixture.

Formula: In the container first put 2 oz (4 tbsp, 59 ml) of vegetable glycerin add 1 oz (2 tbsp, 30 ml) of full-strength tea tree oil. Seal and shake the mixture, then add 1 oz (2 tbsp, 30 ml) of water. Tightly seal the container. Finally shake the mixture vigorously.

Test to see if the tea tree oil is evenly dispersed in the glycerin. Place the mixture on a flat surface or counter top and let it stand for a couple of minutes. If a thin film or drops of the oil start appearing on the surface, add more glycerin and shake until the oil is fully dissolved. The mixture is okay and the tea tree is fully dispersed in it if the container looks uniformly cloudy.

Label the container *Water Soluble Concentrated Tea Tree Oil Mixture in a Glycerin base – Oral, Inhalation & Topical*

Note   The procedures used to create water-soluble solutions of tea tree oil are the same ones used for most essential oils. They are the basis of numerous aromatherapy products such a bath and beauty aids, air sprays and skin care products.

Keep a bottle of the water soluble tea tree oil and glycerin based mixture on hand at all times. It is very beneficial for those minor scraps, cuts and burns that occur when children play or around the kitchen.

Money saving tip. In most cases a 15% solution of tea tree oil is as effective as a full-strength tea tree oil solution. To make a 15% solution, all you do to any of the above mixtures, where 1/2 oz (1 tbsp, 15 ml) of pure tea tree oil is used, is add 3 oz (6 tbsp, 89 ml) of aloe vera gel, water, herbal tea or any combination of these liquids up to 3 oz (6 tbsp, 89 ml). This is close enough to 15% to be beneficial.

For a smaller amount of water soluble glycerin blend, mix 30 drops of pure tea tree oil with 1 tsp (1/6 oz, 5 ml) of glycerin and 1 tsp (1/6 oz, 5 ml) aloe vera, herbal tea or water.

For larger amounts of water soluble glycerin blends, the ratio is approximately 1 part pure tea tree oil to 6 parts of the other base liquids.

General guidelines for tea tree oil uses

For the following applications, full-strength tea tree oil is used, unless otherwise stated. If you use one of the water soluble solutions you may increase the amount of pure tea tree oil to enhance the therapeutic effects. In those cases use the lesser amount of full strength tea tree oil drops recommended for the application.

Bathing – Whole Body

To bath water, add 8-12 drops if pure tea tree oil and/or 1 tsp (1/6 oz, 5 ml) of a water soluble mixture to the running water, when filling the bath. By hand, stir into the water. Bath and relax in the water for 10 minutes or longer.

Bathing – Hands or Feet

To a shallow bath or bowl of warm water, add 5 - 8 drops of pure tea tree oil and/or 1 tsp (1/6 oz, 5 ml) of a water soluble mixture. Soak feet or hands for 5 to 10 minutes.

Bathing – Lower Body (sitz bath)

To a shallow bath add 1 tsp (1/6 oz, 5 ml) of the water soluble concentrated tea tree oil mixture in a glycerin or grain alcohol base. If the problem is acute add 3-6 more drops of pure tea tree oil to the water. Mix thoroughly. Sit in the bath for 5 to 10 minutes. Bathe the affected areas thoroughly.

Good for vaginal, genitourinary infections and other lower body uses.

Air borne methods: Vaporization/Spray Mister/Atomizers

Many methods are available for dispersing tea tree oil into the air. Vaporization makes tea tree oil gaseous by heating it up. To vaporize the oil, you can use an electric diffuser, room vaporizer, facial steamer, ceramic or metal essential oil heating ring you put on a light bulb. With electric appliances it is important to follow the operating directions that come with the unit.

Another option is a small bowl of hot water placed on a gentle source of heat such as a radiator. All you have to do is add a few drops of tea tree oil to the water.

These are effective ways to prevent the spread of contagious illness, disinfect a sick room or get the tea tree oil into a specific area. Some of the air borne methods of dispersing tea tree oil also repel insects and reduce mold.

Atomizers or a spray mister use water and tea tree oil or tea tree oil in a water soluble base to shot out a fine spray mist without heating the contents. Shake container vigorously, before using.

Depending on the conditions being treated you may use the premixed 'Water Soluble Concentrated Tea Tree Oil Mixture in a Grain Alcohol Base' or the 'Water Soluble Concentrated Tea Tree Oil Mixture in a Glycerin Base' as previously described in this chapter. If a condition persists, add a few more drops of tea tree oil to the mixture.

Creams

Here is a simple cream for the skin. Add 6-10 drops of pure tea tree oil to 1/4 cup (2 oz, 60 ml) of KY jelly or vitamin E ointment. Apply as needed.

Compress/Poultice

A compress is a pad of folded cloth, often wet or medicated, that is applied to the skin. It may be hot or cold.

For a quick and easy disinfectant compress, dip a cotton ball, face cloth or soft fabric such as flannel into a bowl of steaming hot or ice cold water containing 3-6 drops of tea tree oil.

A poultice is a hot, soft, moist mass applied to a sore part of the body.

To make a poultice stir in 3-6 drops of tea tree oil to a kaolin or clay base. Make sure to mix it well. Warm the mixture. Particularly beneficial in drawing pus from infected areas such as infected splinters, boils and abscesses.

Dental Care and Gargling

Two quick methods are:

For gargling mix 4-6 drops of pure tea tree oil in a glass of warm water. Then gargle until you have thoroughly rinsed the mouth.

Create your own tea tree oil toothpaste. Blend 6-8 drops of pure tea tree oil with 1 tbsp (1/2 oz, 15 ml) of your favorite toothpaste. You can also put a drop of pure tea tree oil on top of the toothpaste on your toothbrush, or on a finger and rub it onto your gums and teeth before brushing. Tea tree oil does not taste very good, but the toothpaste will help mask its taste. To enhance the benefits of tea tree oil toothpaste, a good electric toothbrush is definitely worth investing in.

These methods can help soften and reduce plaque formation, treat bad breath, mouth ulcers, sore throats, gingivitis, gum infections, etcetera.

Direct/Neat

Direct or neat means unmixed and undiluted pure tea tree oil is applied to the area being treated. Use it straight from the bottle. Put a drop on your finger, a cotton swab or cotton ball. Apply directly to treat burns, cold sores, cuts, open wounds, etcetera.

Caution   Even though tea tree oil is non-toxic, some people find pure tea tree oil to be irritating to the skin. Usually this is because the tea tree oil has too high a para-cymene content or an individual is sensitive to one of the oil's components. If irritation occurs bathe the area in cold water. In the future you may want to dilute the tea tree oil in water or use a 15% tea tree oil water soluble mixture. Another choice is to try a different brand of tea tree oil. The final alternative is to discontinue use altogether. Speak with your health care provider or practitioner if you are unsure about what you should do.

Douche or Sitz Bath

A douche is a jet of liquid applied externally or internally to the body.

To a bowl of warm water add 1 tsp (1/6 oz, 5 ml) of the water soluble tea tree oil mixture in a glycerin or grain alcohol base – see Water-soluble Tea Tree Oil Mixtures in this chapter. If the problem is acute, add 3-6 more drops of pure tea tree oil to the bowl of water. Mix thoroughly. Use as a douche or to bathe the affected area.

A sitz bath is a therapeutic bath in which only the hips and buttocks are immersed. Some use it in conjunction with a douche to bathe the external genitalia. It increases the effectiveness of the treatment, particularly in extreme or prolonged cases of infection. Discontinue use if irritation occurs and consult with a health practitioner.

To a shallow bath add 1 tbsp (1/2 oz, 15 ml) of the water soluble concentrated tea tree oil mixture in a glycerin base—see Water-soluble Tea Tree Oil Mixtures in this chapter. If the problem is acute add 3-6 more drops of pure tea tree oil to the water. Mix thoroughly. Sit in the bath and thoroughly bathe the affected area using this mixture.

Inhalation

Inhalation means breathing in the vapors, mist or steam. Steam inhalation creates a facial sauna. Whether at room temperature or with steam, tea tree oil is a useful addition to your health care needs.

On a tissue or handkerchief put up to 6 drops of tea tree oil. Inhale throughout the day. At night put 2-3 drops onto your pillow and just bellow where you rest your nose. Tea tree oil is non-staining and generally not irritating. This is beneficial for treating colds, flu, etcetera.

For respiratory problems, put up to 6 drops of pure tea tree oil into a bowl of steaming water or add 2-3 drops to the water in the reservoir of a facial steamer. The heat releases the oil into the air. Use a towel to cover your head and the bowl. Close your eyes. Breathe deeply for 5 to 15 minutes.

In addition to treating respiratory problems, steam saunas are an effective way to clear the skin of acne, unblock pores, treat blackheads, etcetera.

Massage

Massage is touching the skin by rubbing or kneading a part of the body. It stimulates the circulation, aids the lymphatic system and in addition increases the production and release of oxytocin, a powerful natural healing hormone in the body. Combine that with the beneficial properties of tea tree oil and you have a powerful therapeutic combination.

When using tea tree oil for massage, mix it with a light vegetable oil as a carrier base. Different base oils have different properties. Cold pressed unadulterated oils are preferred. They do not contain the harsh chemicals that are used in the processing of many oils, nor are they processed at high temperatures that may weaken or destroy some or all of the beneficial properties of these base oils.

Try the following cold pressed oils: jojoba, sweet almond oil, corn or grapeseed. Soya oil, sunflower, apricot kernel, avocado, hazelnut, peanut and olive oil can be used. Jojoba oil is a liquid wax and does not go rancid. The other oils can go rancid. To prolong their shelf life, add a little wheat germ oil, which has vitamin E and anti-oxidant properties.

How much tea tree oil you add depends on the surface area and problem you are dealing with. In the case of muscular aches and pains you may want to make a 5 percent dilution of tea tree oil to base oil. Generally a concentration of 2 -3 percent is sufficient for most needs.

Guidelines—2 1/2 percent tea tree oil dilution by volume:

to: 1 tsp (1/6 oz, 5 ml) base oil add 2-3 drops tea tree oil
   1 tbsp (1/2 oz, 15 ml) base oil add 7-8 drops tea tree oil
   1/4 cup (2 oz, 59 ml) base oil add 30 drops tea tree oil

   20 drops = 1/30 oz = 1 ml

For massage purposes, a little bit of tea tree oil diluted in a carrier base oil, will give a lot of coverage. Shake the contents vigorously before each application to ensure the oil is fully dispersed in it. Apply to the affected area 2 to 4 times daily at the beginning, then reduce to twice daily.

Carrier (base) Oil Type, Benefits and Percentage to Use

The vegetable oils used should be cold pressed since this process does not use chemical agents in the manufacturing. A 10% dilution means that an oil can be added to the base oil up to 10% of the total volume of base oil.

A 100% dilution indicates that you can use it for all or any portion of the carrier base oil volume you desire.

Base carrier oils that best match each condition are indicated in the recommendations for specific tea tree applications. For example, sweet almond oil is good for inflammation, so that would be a base carrier oil of choice to mix with tea tree oil for conditions such as bursitis, carpal tunnel syndrome, repetitive strain syndrome, etcetera. The guidelines for the skin types, what each base oil is effective on and the maximum percentage according to volume of the base oil, are supplied below.

Note   If you or a child are allergic to peanuts, properly processed oils such as sweet almond, hazelnut or peanut oils do not contain the protein that causes these allergic reactions and should not pose a problem. To be on the safe side, speak to your doctor, allergists or health care provider if in doubt.

Sweet Almond Oil
Relieves itching, dryness, soreness and inflammation
All skin types – can be used 100% as base oil

Apricot Kernel Oil
Good for prematurely aged, dry, inflamed and sensitive skin
All skin types – can be used as 100% base oil

Avocado Pear Oil
Good for dehydrated and dry skin, eczema
All skin types – use as 10% dilution with other base oil

Borage Seed Oil
Good for heart disease, multiple sclerosis, menopausal problems, PMS, psoriasis and eczema, prematurely aged skin. Stimulates and regenerates skin.
All skin types – use as 10% dilution with other base oil

Carrot Oil – also an essential oil
Good for itching, premature aging, psoriasis and eczema. Rejuvenating and reduces scarring.
Do not use undiluted – use as 10% dilution with other base oil

Corn Oil
Soothing on all skin types
All skin types – can be used as 100% base oil

Evening Primrose Oil
Good for heart disease, multiple sclerosis, menopausal problems, PMS, psoriasis and eczema, prematurely aged skin. Helps prevent premature aging of skin
All skin types – use as 10% dilution with other base oil

Grapeseed Oil
All skin types – can be used as 100% base oil

Hazelnut Oil
Mildly astringent action
All skin types – can be used as 100% base oil

Jojoba Oil
Good for acne, hair care, inflamed skin, psoriasis and eczema. It is highly penetrative. This is the oil used by Native Americans for smooth, soft and healthy skin.
All skin types – use as 10% dilution with other base oil

Olive Oil (Extra virgin)
Good for cosmetics, hair care, rheumatic conditions. Soothing.
All skin types – use as 10% dilution with other base oil

Peanut Oil (Arachis Nut)
All skin types – can be used as 100% base oil

Safflower Oil
> All skin types – can be used as 100% base oil

Sesame Oil
> Good for arthritis, eczema, psoriasis, rheumatism
> All skin types – use as 10% dilution with other base oil

Soya Oil
> All skin types – can be used as 100% base oil

Sunflower Oil
> All skin types – can be used as 100% base oil

Wheat germ Oil
> Good for eczema, psoriasis, prematurely aged skin
> All skin types – use as 10% dilution with other base oil

Shampoo and Hair Care

Commercial tea tree oil shampoo usually has a 2 1/2 -4 per cent concentration of tea tree oil. To make your own shampoo, buy a neutral pH balanced shampoo and add tea tree oil to it. Add 20 drops (1/30 oz, 1 ml) of pure tea tree oil for each ounce (2 tbsp, 30 ml) of shampoo.

Here's an example for a larger volume: Add 80 drops (2/15 oz, 4 ml) of tea tree oil to 1/2 cup (4 oz, 118 ml) of shampoo. Shake vigorously before each use.

The benefits of tea tree oil shampoo include prevention and a cure for dandruff, head lice, etcetera. It helps clean out hair follicle roots, is stimulating and maintains healthy growth.

A good scalp rub is a grain alcohol based mixture of 6-8 drops of pure tea tree oil added to 1/2 cup (4 oz, 118 ml) of vodka. Shake vigorously before each use. This is one of the formulations used to help get rid of fleas and lice. Caution should be exercised with alcohol based mixtures, on sensitive skin.

Skin Treatments: Creams, Gels, Lotions, Masks and Oils

For skin creams, gels, masks and oils use the proportions listed below. It is recommended that non-allergenic products be used as a carrier base. Many scent free products mask the actual scent of the product with another scent. The better a carrier base product is, the greater the likelihood it will enhance the beneficial aspects of tea tree oil.

To make a light water based lotion, a rough rule of thumb is to use a ratio of 4 parts distilled water to 1 part tea tree oil. For example, for every ounce of distilled water use 1/4 of an ounce of pure tea tree oil (to 4 tsp of distilled water add 1 tsp of tea tree oil. To 100 ml of distilled water add 25 ml tea tree oil). Shake vigorously, each time before you use it. Refer to the section on *Three Water-soluble Tea Tree Oil Mixtures* at the beginning of this chapter, for a better understanding of water soluble mixtures, their uses and general benefits. Different health conditions and beauty uses require different applications and solutions of tea tree oil to maximize the benefits.

In terms of oils, different base oils have different properties. Cold pressed unadulterated oils are preferred. They do not contain the harsh chemicals that are used in the processing of many oils, nor are they processed at high temperatures which may destroy some of the beneficial properties of these base oils. The following can be used for 100 percent of the carrier base oil volume and are okay for all skin types: sweet almond oil, apricot kernel, corn, grapeseed, hazelnut, peanut, safflower, soya and sunflower oils.

Jojoba oil is highly penetrative and does not go rancid, since it is a liquid wax. The other oils may go rancid. To prolong their shelf life, add a little wheat germ oil, which has vitamin E and anti-oxidant properties. You may store them in the refrigerator to prolong their shelf life. If they get cloudy like olive oil does when stored in a refrigerator, warm them up in your hand before applying to the body.

How much tea tree oil you add depends on the surface area and the problem you are dealing with. In some cases you may want to make a 5, 15 or 20 percent dilution of tea tree oil to the carrier base. Generally a concentration of 2-3 percent is sufficient for most creams, gels, lotions, masks and oils.

Guidelines—2 1/2 percent tea tree oil dilution:

to: 1 tsp (1/6 oz, 5 ml) base oil   add 2-3 drops tea tree oil
       1 tbsp (1/2 oz, 15 ml) base oil   add 7-8 drops tea tree oil
       1/4 cup (2 oz, 59 ml) base oil   add 30 drops tea tree oil

Guidelines—5 percent tea tree oil dilution:

to: 1 tsp (1/6 oz, 5 ml) base   add 5 drops tea tree oil
          1 tbsp (1/2 oz, 15 ml) base   add 15 drops tea tree oil
          1/4 cup (2 oz, 59 ml) base   add 59 drops tea tree oil

Guidelines—15 percent tea tree oil dilution:

to: 1 tsp (1/6 oz, 5 ml) base   add 15 drops tea tree oil
          1 tbsp (1/2 oz, 15 ml) base   add 45 drops tea tree oil
          1/4 cup (2 oz, 59 ml) base   add just under 2 tsp tea
                                           tree oil

Guidelines—20 percent tea tree oil dilution:

to: 1 tsp (1/6 oz, 5 ml) base   add 20 drops tea tree oil
          1 tbsp (1/2 oz, 15 ml) base   add 60 drops tea tree oil
          1/4 cup (2 oz, 59 ml) base   add 2 1/3 tsp tea tree oil

       20 drops   =   1/30 oz   =   1 ml

Shake or mix the contents before using. The number of applications, what dilutions, when and how to use these products varies with the application.

Special note regarding health care use options

In many situations, tea tree oil may not be sufficient to deal with the underlying cause of an illness or disease. In those cases it is wise to combine tea tree oil use with other approaches such as acupuncture, counseling, dietary changes, herbal medicine, homeopathy, nutritional supplementation, stress reducing methods, traditional medicine, relaxation techniques, other essential oils, etcetera.

A very powerful healing combination is the use of tea tree oil to complement traditional allopathic medicine. Give your health care provider a copy of this book, to aid them in your mutually beneficial quest for health and healing. This can be a very powerful healing combination.

CHAPTER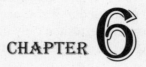

Summary of Properties and Uses— Safety Data, Standards of Quality and Storage Precautions

Safety data

Research and findings since the beginning of the twentieth century indicate tea tree oil is generally non-irritating, non-sensitizing and non-toxic. For all intents and purposes, its almost neutral pH balance makes it neither alkaline nor acidic. It is non-corrosive, non-staining and easy to use. It maintains its clear properties when mixed in water.

Tea tree oil only destroys the pathogens, microorganisms capable of causing disease, not the healthy skin tissue. People with extremely sensitive skin, may need to use a dilution of pure oil or avoid it.

In 1992 a case was cited by J. Weyland and A. de Groot in the *Natural Database U.K. Aromatherapy* about a patient with atopic dermatitis.[17] The tea tree oil was put directly on the skin. The patient's condition worsened. Next, oral ingestion was tried, and the condition only worsened. Further investigation found the allergen to be the cineole content of the tea tree oil.

In 1989, the *International Journal of Aromatherapy*[18] reported the case of a boy with athlete's foot, being treated with tea tree oil which further aggravated his condition. Speculation about the patient's allergic reaction indicated a need for further research.[19]

To determine if you are highly sensitive or allergic to tea tree

oil, do a *patch test* before using it for the first time. The procedure is simple, you put a couple of drops of tea tee oil on the
back of your wrist and leave it there for an hour, or better yet for
12 hours or overnight. If skin irritation occurs, wash the area
with cold water. If you are concerned, see your doctor and do
the 'patch test' under his supervision. When irritation occurs
due to the patch test, then only use tea tree oil in diluted form or
avoid using it or try another brand.

Caution   Because of their high levels of concentration, *all essential oils* require special care and use with babies, young
children, pregnant or lactating women. Even though
tea tree oil is considered non-toxic, it should not be
used undiluted on children under 18 months old.
During pregnancy always dilute the tea tree oil to half
its usual concentration. As with all essential oils, tea
tree oil should not be taken internally, unless you are
under medical supervision. There may be cause for
concern if a young child swallows a teaspoon (1/6 oz,
5 ml) or more of tea tree oil.

Pure tea tree oil, because of its concentration, can be irritating and generally should be used very sparingly or not at all
on small animals, cats or dogs. In September 1994, the *Small
Animal Medicine and Surgery* veterinary journal, reported that
the National Animal Poison Control Center indicated *Melaleuca
toxicosis,* when high doses of undiluted tea tree oil were topically
applied, to treat skin conditions in cats and dogs. Within 2 to 8
hours of use, the following symptoms were noted: weakness,
depression, poor coordination and muscle tremors. Within 3 to
4 days the reactions disappeared. Rarely, if ever should high
doses of undiluted tea tree oil be used on pets. When recommended to treat difficult conditions, use sparingly, with care and
avoid the eye area. Watch your pet for any adverse reaction. If
one occurs stop treatment with undiluted tea tree oil immediately. Generally a 15 percent tea tree oil dilution is preferred and
is usually just as effective as pure tea tree oil.

In summary pure tea tree oil is generally non-toxic and safe
to use. Pure undiluted tea tree oil is not recommended for
babies, young children, pregnant or lactating women and some

pets. Consult your health practitioner first if in doubt. If skin irritation problems occur, try another brand. Australian and International Standards Organization (ISO) parameters for the pharmaceutical grade of pure tea tree oil, are helping to insure a consistent quality of pure tea tree oil for therapeutic uses.

Standards of Quality

Increasing international interest and scientific research into the safety and multitude of uses for tea tree oil is causing substantial growth in the markets for consumer and commercial uses of tea tree oil products. Government agencies and international associations are getting involved in monitoring and regulating the industry.

Under the Food and Drug Administration's (FDA) labeling regulations, synthetic tea tree oils cannot be labeled as pure. However, pure tea tree oil can be a blend from different batches. This has resulted in identifying some suppliers who are using 'adulterated' or 'bogus' oil and bringing pressure to bear upon them, from within the industry.

New standards of quality replaced the Australian AS 2782-1985 standard set in 1985. The AS 2782-1985 standard requires a terpinen-4-ol of greater than 30 percent and a cineole content of less than 15 per cent. The International Standards Organization officially adopted a new Australian standard (ISO 4730), which replaces the old standard. The new standard tests for 40 components and still requires a terpinen-4-ol content of greater than 30 percent and a cineole content of less than 15 per cent. The American Tea Tree Association (ATTA) checks the purity and quality of tea tree oil imported into America.

The criteria for the ISO Standard 4370 pharmaceutical grade are as follows: tea tree oil must be steam distilled from the Melaleuca alternifolia, Melaleuca linarifolia, or Melaleuca dissitiflora species of the Myrtacceae plant family. Other species are not as highly regarded, since they do not have the same antimicrobial benefits, nor have they been in use as long as the tea tree oil from Melaleuca alternifolia plants.

For effective therapeutic results, it is important to get a pharmaceutical grade of tea tree oil. Make sure the label states the source of the tea tree oil is the Melaleuca alternifolia tree and the supplier is a reputable one. If in doubt, write to the supplier or call their consumer information line. Request they send you a copy of the testing done on the batch you are purchasing.

There are many grades of tea tree oil. Up to now, we have only discussed the pharmaceutical grade for human and animal use. Standard and industrial grades, for non-therapeutic products, contain between 30-35% terpinen-4-ol and up to 8% cineole. Both industrial and standard grades are used for disinfectants, floor detergents, fungus and mold killers, as well as in air conditioning and air venting systems. Hospitals overseas use these grades to help reduce the incidence of mold in the hospital.

Storage

Essential oils are prone to rapid deterioration if stored improperly. This is due to oxidation when exposed to air. In addition exposure to sunlight, extremes of heat or cold can cause decline in the beneficial properties of an essential oil.

In tea tree oil, exposure to air causes the active microbial agent, terpinen-4-ol, to decrease. Technically the gamma-terpinene content decreases and the para-cymene content increases. Generally tea tree oil is hardy and does not easily suffer a significant loss of potency when exposed to air, heat or light. When stored properly it has a shelf life of approximately three years, and has been known to stay potent much longer. Proper storage is important to prevent tea tree oil from losing its bactericidal properties.

Six points to remember when storing and using undiluted pure tea tree oil:

- Store in an airtight dark-glass containers.**
- Store away from heat or extreme cold.
- Store away from light.
- Store in a dry cool place.
- Keep out of reach from children and pets.
- Make sure bottle is properly labeled.

**In certain instances, such as diluted mixtures or when small amounts of oil are thoroughly mixed into a base, a clear plastic container is suitable.

Caution: Pure tea tree oil can dissolve some plastics. Be careful on wood and plastic based finishes it comes in contact with.

The tea tree oil money saving home healer quick shopping list

Use this shopping list for the ingredients and items to use with tea tree oil. Most of them are available in pharmacies, drug stores, supermarkets and health food stores or already in your home. The majority of these products have multiple uses and long shelf lives, so they should not go to waste. In many cases they are biodegradable and are the basis of numerous, more expensive manufactured products.

The benefits include less wasteful consumer packaging. Make sure you read the product labels, use and store them correctly. In many cases pure tea tree oil is used to enhance and boost the benefits of these and other products. Use this basic shopping list in combination with pure tea tree oil to create many of the health, beauty, plant, pet and cleaning aids you want. You will save money, be kinder to our planet and importantly live in a less stressful and healthier environment.

Tea Tree Oil (Melaleuca alternifolia)

Distilled Witch Hazel (Hamamelis water)

Glycerin – preferably vegetable

Distilled water or use cold boiled water

Rubbing alcohol (Isopropyl alcohol)

Light mineral oil

Wheat germ oil or encapsulated wheat germ oil

Epsom salts (magnesium sulfate heptahydrate) Bath salts

Calamine lotion (Active ingredients: Zinc oxide, calamine, calcium hydroxide. Inactive ingredients: bebtonite, glycerin, imidurea, water)

Zinc ointment (Active ingredient 15% zinc oxide. Inactive ingredients: anhydrous lanolin, cetostearyl alcohol, paraffin, white petroleum)

Ihle's Paste (Active ingredients: Zinc oxide. Inactive ingredients: Lanolin, starch, white petroleum)

Friar's Balsam (Active ingredients: Benzoin, aloe, storax, Tolu balsam. Inactive ingredients: Alcohol)

Eucalyptus oil

1 bottle high proof grain alcohol, such as vodka.

Amber or dark colored glass jars and labels

Vaporizer or pot for boiling water

Soft cloth or face cloth

Cotton balls

Cotton swabs

Sterile gauze bandages

1 light vegetable oil. Preferably cold pressed, meaning no harsh chemicals or high temperatures are used to extract and refine the oil, thereby destroying much if not all of its healing properties. This may affect their shelf life, but if you are using the oil for healing, you want the very best. A little goes a long way.

The best choice for a base oil, depends on the problem being treated. For the base oil choose cold pressed, not chemically extracted or heat processed oils. Good general use choices include sweet almond oil, grapeseed, corn, peanut, soya and sunflower oil. Jojoba is a wax, so it does not go rancid and it is also highly penetrative. Other vegetable oils have varying shelf lifes. Cold Pressed Virgin Olive Oil lasts the longest of the edible cooking oils, about 2 years. To extend the shelf life of a cold pressed oil, store it in the refrigerator.

In a class all its own! Cold pressed virgin olive oil has so many known and potential therapeutic properties and uses in food preparation that it should be a staple in your kitchen. Whereas most oils have little or no taste, olive oil's strong flavor offers a hidden cost and weight reduction benefit. You only need to use 2/3 as much of it in cooking and salad recipes as you would use of other cooking oils.

CONGRATULATIONS!

Now you are ready to save money and enhance your life and that of those around you, using this miraculous essential oil. If you find a benefit or new way to use tea tree oil, please share it with the authors of this book. Contact information to write them is in the back of the book. If your comments are used, you will be acknowledged in future editions of *The Tea Tree Oil Bible*. Good luck and good health!

CHAPTER **7**

Health Uses for Tea Tree Oil
—from A to Z

Abscesses • Aches and Pains – Muscular • Acne • AIDS – see Immune System • Arthritis • Athlete's Foot • Bad Breath – Halitosis – Mouth and Gum Infections • Balanitis • Barber's Rash • Bee Stings • Blackheads • Blocked Nasal Passages • Boils • Bronchitis • Bronchial Congestion • Bruises and Bumps • Bunions • Burns and Sunburn • Bursitis • Calluses • Canker Sores – oral • Candida Albicans • Carbuncles • Carpal Tunnel Syndrome • Chapped Lips • Chicken pox • Chiggers • Chilblains • Chronic Fatigue – see Immune System • Calvus • Colds/Fever • Cold Sores • Congestion • Coral Cuts • Corns • Coughs • Crabs • Cradle Cap • Cramps • Cuticles • Cuts and Abrasions • Cracked Dry Skin • Cystitis/Urethritis • Dandruff • Dental Plaque • Dermatitis • Dhobi Itch • Diaper Rash • Diabetic Gangrene • Ear Infections • Ear Wax • Earaches • Eczema • Emphysema • Fever • Flu • Foot Odor • Fungal Infections • Furuncle • Genital Herpes • Genitourinary Infections • Gingivitis – Mouth and Gum Infections • Gout • Head Lice • Head Cold • Herpes • Hives • Hemorrhoids • Hepatitis • Immune System – to Strengthen • Impetigo • Ingrown Toenails • Insect Bites • Itching • Leeches and Ticks • Leg Ulcers • Leucorrhoea • Lice (Pediculosis) • Measles • Moniliasis • Mouth and Gum Infections • Mouth Ulcers • Muscular Aches and Pains • Nails (Infected) • Nettle Rash • Nipples (Sore) • Ovarian Cysts • Paronychia • Piles • Pimples • Plantar Warts • Poison Ivy and Poison Oak • Prickly Heat •

Pruritis • Psoriasis • Respiratory Tract Infections • Rheumatism • Ringworm • Salpingitis • Scabies • Shaver's Rash • Shingles • Sinusitis • Sore Nipples • Sore Throat • Splinters • Sprains • Stiff Muscles • Stiff Neck • Styes • Sunburn and Burns • Surgery – uses in • Sweaty Feet • Thrush • Ticks and Leeches • Tinea cruris – check out pedis, barbae • Tooth Ache • Tonsillitis • Ulcers: Varicose and Tropical • Urethritis • Vaginal Infections • Veruccae • Warts • Wounds • Zona

Abscesses

An abscess is due to an infection of a sebaceous gland. This results in an inflammation of the skin and localized painful swelling. It is caused when the body is stressed or run-down. As the result of a blood disorder. At times of hormonal upheaval. It is an indication that the body is in need of purification.

Medical research indicates tea tree oil is a superb treatment for abscesses. It penetrates the skin, fighting the infection and breaking down the pus without the need to break the skin.

Recommendations

Eat lots of fresh fruits and vegetables. Avoid stimulants. Drink plenty of water and an herbal tea tree infusion – either hot or as a refreshing ice cold tea. Tea tree oil is an immune system stimulant and can help prevent, maintain or help the healing of an abscess from within. It should be done in conjunction with one of the following approaches:

As soon as an abscess appears, start treatment. Do not wait for it to burst. Apply pure tea tree oil onto your finger or a cotton swab and dab it onto the abscessed area, making sure you cover it completely. Repeat 2 to 3 times a day. Continue until all signs of abscess are gone.

If an external abscess has already formed, mix 3-4 drops of tea tree oil into a warm clay poultice, then apply it onto the affected area. Leave the poultice on it for a half hour. This draws the pus or liquid from the abscess. Then gently bathe the affected area with a clean cloth.

Another choice is to apply a warm face cloth that has been

soaked in a water soluble alcohol based tea tree oil solution, onto the abscess. Let it sit for a few minutes. Next put 1-2 drops of pure tea tree oil onto the abscess. Repeat this 2 to 4 times a day.

In severe cases, with external abscesses, cover it with a gauze soaked in tea tree oil for 10 to 12 hours. Seek medical attention if there is no improvement.

As a general disinfectant method, add 8 -12 drops of tea tree oil or a water soluble tea tree oil solution, to bath water, and soak in it for 10-20 minutes.

Abrasions – see Cuts

Recommendations

Clean and wash affected area with a soft cloth and warm water. Apply a few drops of pure tea tree oil and a bandage if needed. Repeat several times a day until the skin has healed.

For minor abrasions mix 1-2 drops of pure tea tree oil with some honey and apply to the affected area. Cover with a Band Aid or gauze. Apply and change dressing as needed.

Aches and Pains – Muscular

Muscular aches and pains are a common problem caused by psychological stress or physical over-exertion. Over time the ache or pain causes the muscles to become tight and more painful. Neck and shoulder tension are commonly associated areas where muscular aches and pains tend to reside.

Recommendations

Apply this soothing and healing lotion to the problem area. It is particularly effective for bruises and sprains. Mix 2 tbsp (1 oz, 30 ml) of distilled witch hazel (Hamamelis water) and 15-20 drops of tea tree oil. Shake lotion vigorously before applying to skin. Apply to the affected area. After applying the lotion cover it with a moist soft cloth. Keep area moist until relieved.

Soak in a hot bath. Add 8-12 drops of pure tea tree oil to the hot water when your filling up the bath tub. Stir the water once the tub is full. Soak for 10-20 minutes. The penetrating and pain-killing (analgesic) properties of tea tree oil increase the benefits of the hot bath.

To relieve stiff muscles, mix 2-4 drops of pure tea tree oil with isopropyl alcohol (rubbing alcohol) and rub into the affected area as needed.

Muscular spasms or very tight areas can be relieved by massaging a few drops of pure tee tree oil into the affected area. You can also add a few drops of pure tea tree oil to a hot compress and apply it to the area.

Massage the affected muscular aches and pains areas with this massage oil: Mix 9 drops of pure tea tree oil in 1 tbsp (1/2 oz, 15 ml) of a light cold pressed vegetable oil, such as jojoba, grapeseed, sweet almond, olive, peanut oil. Mix thoroughly. Repeat as often as needed.

Prevention of muscular aches and pains, can be accomplished by massaging a few drops of pure tea tree oil immediately before and just after the strenuous activities.

Acne

Acne is an unsightly skin condition. It is very common during adolescence and during times of hormonal upheaval, such as before and after menstruation and menopause. The condition shows up as greasy and congested skin resulting in a rough surface texture, enlarged pores, pimples, blackheads and spots.

Acne is the result of overactivity of the sebaceous glands. The condition is worsened by lack of proper nutrition, poor diet, not enough exercise or physical activity, poor personal hygiene, stress and emotional factors.

Recommendations

Prevent the condition from spreading and worsening by paying particular attention to personal hygiene. Wash affected area with an hypo-allergenic unscented pH balanced soap or a tea tree oil soap, containing 2 to 5% tea tree oil.

Put undiluted tea tree oil on a cotton swab or your finger and apply directly to the individual spots at night before going to sleep and in the morning. If it is a particularly bad condition apply 4 times the first and second day, then 2 or 3 times for the next three days.

Mix 2-4 drops of tea tree oil with a small amount of beeswax or apply a commercially prepared tea tree oil in a beeswax base to the spots.

Make a 5% dilution of tea tree oil by mixing it with an hypo-allergenic non-greasy cream, gel or lotion. For 1 tbsp (1/2 oz, 15 ml) of base use 15 drops of tea tree oil. For 1/4 cup (2 oz, 60 ml) use 60 drops of essential tea tree oil. Commercially available tea tree ointments are available. Apply as a cleansing and moisturizing agent.

In a container with a top, mix 1/2 cup (4 oz, 118 ml) of distilled water with 30 drops of tea tree oil. Before each use, shake the container vigorously. Make sure to use a clean cloth each time. Bathe the affected areas with the mixture morning and night.

Add 8 to 12 drops of tea tree oil to bath, once it is filled with water. Soak and relax in the bath tub for at least 10 minutes. One advantage of this is that you get a facial steam this way.

Create your own facial sauna. To a bowl of boiling water, add 3 to 5 drops of pure tea tree oil or in a facial steamer add 1-3 drops of tea tree oil to the water in the reservoir. Use a towel to cover your head and the bowl or facial steamer. Let your face enjoy the steam for 8 to 15 minutes. Do this 3 to 5 times a week.

AIDS – see Immune System

Acquired Immune Deficiency Syndrome (AIDS) results in numerous conditions that threaten one's health. To the best of our knowledge no studies have been reported regarding the use of tea tree oil in terms of directly treating AIDS. We have heard positive stories from AIDS patients who have used it to treat some of the conditions listed in this book. We suggest you review the documented benefits of tea tree oil use and share them with your health care practitioner. This can be a powerful tool, to help you deal with the various conditions as they arise.

Healing from the inside out, means using the body's natural wisdom to heal itself. Drink a tea tree oil herbal tea – either hot or as a refreshing ice cold tea. Use a commercially prepared tea tree oil tea. Tea tree oil is an immune system stimulant and may be of some benefit to you.

Caution should be taken, since it is not recommended that you ingest pure tea tree oil due to its high concentration. Speak with your health care practitioner before making your own tea.

Arthritis

Arthritis is characterized by an inflammation and/or pain in a joint or joints. Symptoms include swelling, redness of the skin and impaired motion. Two types of arthritis are: Osteoarthritis which is chronic, involves joints, especially those that are weight-bearing. Rheumatoid arthritis which is chronic, manifested by inflammatory changes in joints which can be crippling. It is a degenerative joint disease.

In young women, there may be a link between the bacteria responsible for chlamydia nonspecific urethritis and their arthritic condition.

The principle benefit tea tree oil offers sufferers is pain relief. In cases where bacteria may be the suspected cause, tea tree oils antibacterial and anti-inflammatory properties appear to be well suited for the situation.

Contributing factors to this condition are emotional conflict, stress, lack of exercise, improper nutrition and poor diet.

Recommendation

Make a massage oil by mixing 18 drops of pure tea tree oil in 1/8 cup (1 oz, 2 tbsp, 30 ml) of a light vegetable carrier oil, such as jojoba, grapeseed or sweet almond oil. It is preferable to use an organically produced vegetable oil, since it nourishes the skin better and is not chemically extracted. Shake or mix the contents before each application. Store the massage oil in a dark bottle, away from sunlight. A little of this massage oil will go a long way! Apply 2 to 4 times daily at the beginning, then reduce to twice daily.

To reduce inflammation, apply a cold compress using a face cloth or flannel cloth upon which you have added a few drops of pure tea tree oil. A cold compress using clay and a few drops of pure tea tree oil mixed into it, is also beneficial.

Bathing. For pain relief add 8 to 12 drops of pure tea tree oil to the bath water when you are filling the bath tub. Relax and enjoy.

Athlete's Foot

Athlete's foot is ringworm, a contagious skin disease caused by a fungus, *Tinea pedis*, of the foot. It is commonly characterized by red, flaky or soggy skin and itching between the toes. The heels and soles can become covered in a white scaly skin. The fungus can also affect fingers and nails.

Usually the affected skin cracks and becomes painful. In such cases the feet should be exposed to air and be allowed to breath as much as and whenever possible. It is highly contagious and usually picked up in schools and changing rooms.

Keep feet area dry by wearing socks and shoes that can breath and release and keep moisture away from the skin. Add a few drops of tea tree oil to the wash water to disinfect socks.

Recommendations

Bath feet with an antifungal soap or tea tree oil soap. Dry feet thoroughly then apply pure tea tree oil [or 15-20 drops of pure tea tree oil mixed with 1 tbsp (1/2 oz, 5 ml) of olive oil]. Massage a few drops of pure tea tree oil into the area affected by the fungus in the morning and before bed . If the condition is chronic, more applications during the day may be required. Continue until condition clears up. You can also add 1 to 2 tbsp of this to your bath water.

Apply this mixture. Mix 1 tbsp (1/2 oz, 15 ml) of isopropyl alcohol and 2 tbsp (1 oz, 30 ml) of pure tea tree oil. Shake vigorously. Let bottle rest on a flat surface for a couple of minutes. If tea tree oil floats to the surface, add more alcohol and shake again until oil is evenly dispersed in the mixture. Store it in a glass bottle and cool place. This quantity will last for quite a while, has many uses and can be used as a disinfectant. You can add 1 to 2 tbsp of this to your bath water.

Soak feet in a shallow bath of 5-10 drops of pure tea tree oil and warm water, for 5-10 minutes each day. Dry feet thoroughly using an absorbent towel and/or a hair dryer.

As a preventative measure add 8 to 12 drops of pure tea tree oil to the bath water when you are filling the bath tub.

Bad Breath (Halitosis) – see Mouth and Gum Infections

Bad breath (Halitosis) is usually caused by poor dental hygiene. Many other factors can affect your breath: gum or tooth decay, poor diet, constipation, throat and nose infections, smoking, indigestion, foreign bacteria in the mouth, etcetera. If bacteria are the cause, tea tree oil is very effective.

Recommendations

Brush your teeth, gums and tongue with a commercially prepared tea tree oil toothpaste or put a drop of pure tree tea oil on your regular brand of toothpaste. A good electric tooth brush, gently applied to the gums, tongue and cheeks as well as the teeth, will reduce your mouths bacterial count.

Gargle with a mouthwash to which you add tea tree oil. Most mouthwashes contain alcohol. Add 6-10 drops of tea tree oil to the mouthwash. The more alcohol content it has, the easier the oil will dissolve and stay evenly dispersed in it. Shake bottle each time before gargling.

Use dental floss. Commercially prepared dental floss with tea tree oil is available or add a drop of pure tea tree oil onto the dental floss. This boosts the antibacterial benefits.

Balanitis – see Candida, Leucorrhoea/Pruritis, Thrush, Vaginal Infections

Balanitis is an irritating fungal infection, caused by *Candida albicans,* affecting the end of the penis. Usually caused by improper personal hygiene or contracted through sexual contact with a women suffering from thrush or a vaginal infection caused by the same fungus. If unnoticed or untreated by the male, they can easily infect their female partner with the fungus.

To avoid reinfection, it is very important that both male and female sexual partners are simultaneously and successfully treated before resuming sexual relations.

Recommendations

Carefully wash the area with a 1% solution of distilled water and Melaleuca oil, making sure to apply it at least 4 times a day. Shake the solution vigorously each time, before application. To make a 1% solution, use the following amounts. To 1 tbsp (1/2 oz, 15 ml) of distilled water add 3 drops of pure tea tree oil. For 1/4 cup (2 oz, 60 ml) of distilled water use 12 drops of pure tea tree oil.

For more severe cases, make a 5% solution, using the following amounts. For 1 tbsp (1/2 oz, 15 ml) of distilled water use 15 drops of pure tea tree oil. For 1/4 cup (2 oz, 60 ml) of distilled water use 60 drops of pure tea tree oil.

Note Due to the extreme sensitivity of tissue in this area, it is important that any increase in skin irritation be carefully monitored under the supervision of a health care practitioner. In really extreme cases they may want to apply pure tea tree oil using the tip of a finger or a cotton swab.

Note For women, see Candida (vaginal fungal infection) and for men and women see Thrush (mouth and throat fungal infection) for recommendations for treatments of infection by the *Candida albicans* organism.

Barber's Rash

Barber's rash is an eruption of small red pimples on the face and neck, caused by the fungal infection *Tinea barbae*. The skin often becomes flaky and sore. It is aggravated by shaving and can be worsened by an outbreak of acne (refer to Acne for treatment suggestions). To sooth, reduce and heal the irritation as well as prevent additional problems, these tea tree oil blends are very beneficial. Avoid using commercial after-shaves or harsh soaps.

Recommendations

Apply this soothing and healing lotion in the morning and at night time. Mix 2 tbsp (1 oz, 30 ml) of distilled witch hazel (Hamamelis water) and 15-20 drops of tea tree oil. Shake lotion vigorously before applying to skin. Apply to the affected area.

Apply 10-15 drops of pure tea tree oil blended with 2 tbsp (1 oz, 30 ml) of aloe vera gel or juice to the affected area. Shake vigorously before each use. Apply in the morning and at night.

Apply this 2% water soluble lotion. put 4 drops of pure tea tree oil in 1 tsp (1/6 oz, 5 ml) of glycerin. Shake vigorously before applying in the morning and at night.

Apply a 15% tea tree oil water soluble glycerin mixture to the skin. To make this 15% solution, mix 30 drops of pure tea tree oil with 1 tsp (1/6 oz, 5 ml) of glycerin and 1 tsp (1/6 oz, 5 ml) aloe vera. For larger amounts of water soluble glycerin mixtures, the ratio is approximately 1 part of tea tree oil to 6 parts of other base liquids. Apply morning and night.

Massage the face with this massage oil: Mix 9 drops of pure tea tree oil in 1 tbsp (1/2 oz, 15 ml) of a light base oil, such as grapeseed or sweet almond oil. Mix thoroughly before applying. Apply in the morning and at night. This massage oil is not recommended for those suffering from oily skin conditions.

Bee Stings

Bee stings are caused by the release of the chemicals from the stinger, that hooks itself just below the surface of the skin. Even though the stinger and bee are separated, the small chemical laden sac at the end of the stinger, keeps pumping the inflammatory chemicals into the body.

If you have an allergic reaction to bee stings, seek medical help immediately. Have your health care provider prescribe an emergency treatment kit.

Do not use tweezers nor squeeze the end of the stinger and withdraw it, this will only cause the stinger's sac to release the irritating chemicals faster into your body. *The first thing one should do is flick the stinger off the body, to stop the continued release of chemicals.*

Recommendations

Apply a drop of pure tea tree oil to the affected area, every four hours or as required.

Add 8 to 12 drops of pure tea tree oil to a bath, while bath tub is filling up with water. Stir water to disperse the oil. Soak and relax in the bath tub for at least 10 minutes.

Apply this soothing and healing lotion. To 2 tbsp (1 oz, 30 ml) of distilled witch hazel (Hamamelis water) add 15-20 drops of tea tree oil. Shake lotion vigorously before applying to skin. Apply 3-4 times daily. Tea tree oil boosts the effectiveness of this lotion and adds protection against infection.

Apply this protective, soothing, healing and drying lotion. To 2 tbsp (1 oz, 30 ml) of calamine lotion add 15-20 drops of tea tree oil (for children use 5 drops), to the affected area. Shake lotion vigorously before applying to skin. Apply 3-4 times daily. Tea tree oil boosts the effectiveness of these lotions and adds protection against infection, especially if the area blisters.

Tea tree oil is an effective insect repellent. For preventative use, apply pure tea tree oil to exposed skin, clothing such as scarves, socks, collars and cuffs of shirts. For larger areas of skin, apply the following oil and tea tree mixture: To 1/8 cup (1 oz, 2 tbsp, 60 ml) of a cold pressed light vegetable carrier oil such as avocado, jojoba, grapeseed, olive, sweet almond oil, etcetera and 15-18 drops of pure tea tree oil. Shake or mix the contents before each application. A little will go a long way. Apply as needed.

Blackheads

Blackheads are dark plugs of dried fatty matter in a pore of the skin. It is an unsightly skin condition, that is very common during adolescence and during times of hormonal upheaval, such as before and after menstruation and menopause.

A blackhead is a very blocked pore, resulting in a solid material in the blocked pore, that causes the surface of the pore to expand. The blackhead is not dirt. Dermatologists aren't exactly sure about what it is, but know it does not result in pimples.

The condition may be worsened by lack of proper nutrition, poor diet, not enough exercise or physical activity, poor personal hygiene, stress and emotional factors.

Recommendations

Pay particular attention to personal hygiene. Wash affected

area with a mild hypo-allergenic scent free soap or non-scented 100% pure glycerin soap.

Put undiluted pure tea tree oil on a cotton swab or your finger and apply directly to the individual spots at night before going to sleep and in the morning. If it is a particularly bad condition apply 4 times the first day and then twice daily for the next three days.

Make a 5% dilution of pure tea tree oil by mixing it with a hypo-allergenic cream, gel or lotion preferably. For 1 tbsp (1/2 oz, 15 ml) of base use 15 drops of pure tea tree oil. For 1/4 cup (2 oz, 60 ml) use 60 drops of pure tea tree oil. Apply as cleansing and moisturizing agents, always use a clean cloth or wash your hands thoroughly each time.

In a container with a top, mix 1/2 cup (4 oz, 118 ml) of distilled water with 30 drops of pure tea tree oil. Before each use, shake the container vigorously. Morning and night bath the affected areas with the mixture, making sure to use a clean cloth each time.

Add 8 to 12 drops (only 5 drops for children) of pure tea tree oil to bath, while bath tub is filling up with water. Stir water to disperse the oil. Soak and relax in the bath tub for at least 10 minutes.

Create your own facial sauna. To a bowl of boiling water, add 3 to 5 drops of pure tea tree oil. Drape a towel over your head and he bowl. Let your face enjoy the steam for 8 to 15 minutes. Then gently wipe your skin with a clean cloth. Do this 3 to 5 times a week.

Boils (Furuncle)

A boil is due to an infection of a sebaceous gland. This results in an inflammation of the skin and localized painful swelling.

Boils appear when the body is stressed or run-down. As the result of a blood disorder. At times of hormonal upheaval.

It is an indication the body is in need of purification.

Medical research indicates tea tree oil is a superb treatment for boils. It penetrates the skin, fighting the infection and breaking down the pus without the need to break the skin.

Recommendations

Eat lots of fresh fruits and vegetables. Avoid stimulants. Drink plenty of water and a tea tree oil herbal tea – either hot or as a refreshing ice cold tea.

Healing from the inside out, means using the bodies natural wisdom to heal itself. Drink a tea tree oil herbal tea – either hot or as a refreshing ice cold tea. Use a commercially prepared tea tree herbal tea. The essential oil from the tea tree is an immune system stimulant and may help prevent or heal a boil from within. It is not recommended that you ingest pure tea tree essential oil since it is so highly concentrated. Drinking a commercially prepared tea tree herbal preparation, should be done in conjunction with one of the following approaches:

As soon as a boil appears, start treatment. Do not wait for it to burst. Apply pure tea tree oil using your finger or a cotton swab and dab it onto the affected area, making sure you cover it completely. Repeat 2 to 3 times a day. Continue until all signs of the boil are gone.

If an external boil has formed, apply pure tea tree oil to the area and cover with a coating of a beeswax or good hand cream to seal in the oil. You can apply a warm clay poultice containing 3-4 drops of tea tree oil to the boil. Give it a half hour to draw the pus/liquid, then gently bathe the affected area with a clean cloth.

Apply a warm face cloth that has been soaked in tea tree oil. Then dab the boil with tea tree oil straight from the bottle. Repeat this 2-3 times daily. (After each use of the cloth, make sure to disinfect it by adding a few drops of tea tree oil to your laundry with the detergent to avoid transmission of problem causing bacteria.)

If the boil is severe, cover it with a gauze soaked in tea tree oil for 12 hours. If there is no improvement, get medical advice.

Add 8-12 drops of tea tree oil to the bath water, stir vigorously then soak in it for 10 to 20 minutes.

Bronchitis

Bronchitis, an inflammation of the bronchial tubes, is usually accompanied by coughing and mucus congestion. Bronchitis is either acute or chronic.

The acute variety is short term in nature. It may start with a sore throat or cold. This may develop into a fever lasting a few days.

The chronic variety is long-term and no fever develops. The following conditions may aggravate it: Smoking, second hand smoke, air pollution, a damp climate, improper diet – such as too many dairy products and poor nutrition.

It is important to note that bronchitis may lead to complications. The young, elderly and chronically ill should seek medical help as soon as possible, if the condition gets worse.

Tea tree oil can combat the infection, ease the coughing, help the lungs rid themselves of mucus and reduce the fever. In addition it reinforces the body's immune system and prevents the spread of the infection.

Recommendations

As soon as the condition occurs, start steam inhalation to help prevent the infection from developing any further and to soothe coughing. To a bowl of steaming hot water add 5 drops of pure tea tree oil and inhale for 5 to 10 minutes. If you want to capture more of the steam, drape a towel over your head and the bowl. Make sure the table and bowl are very stable and secure. Be very careful not to spill any of the hot water and burn or scald yourself. If using a facial steamer, add 1-2 drops of pure tea tree oil to the water in the reservoir and follow the directions above.

Drink plenty of water and a tea tree herbal tea – either hot or as a refreshing ice cold tea. Hot is better in terms of helping to break up the mucus. The drink may help stimulate your compromised immune system. Use a commercially prepared tea tree herbal tea. It is an immune system stimulant and may help. It is not recommended that you ingest pure tea tree oil.

Take a hot bath. Put 8-12 drops of pure tea tree oil into the bath water. This encourages your body to sweat, which is its natural reaction to fever. The effect is similar to doing steam inhalation. If feverish, especially if the body's temperature is high, use cool water in the bath.

Massage the back, chest and throat with a blend of 2.5 per cent tea tree oil. As a base use 1 tsp (5 ml) of a light oil such as jojoba, grapeseed or sweet almond oil, or a good hand cream or skin lotion and add 3 drops of pure tea tree oil. If you plan to frequently massage the back, chest and throat use 1 tbsp (15 ml) of the base oil and add 9 drops of pure tea tree oil to it.

Inhalation using a vaporizer, is very beneficial. Put 5 drops of pure tea tree oil into the water of your vaporizer at home. This is especially beneficial in the bedroom at night.

Apply a warm wet face cloth, to which you add 4-5 drops of pure tea tree oil, onto the chest. Very helpful for bronchial congestion and emphysema.

On a handkerchief or Kleenex tissue put a few drops of pure tea tree oil for inhalation during the day.

Wash hands thoroughly using a tea tree oil soap with triclosan as an active ingredient. Laboratory testing shows it destroys the harmful bacteria like Strep., E. coli, Salmonella, Staph and viruses. This helps prevent the transmission of disease causing agents.

Note   Consult your family health care provider, if condition worsens, or you are in doubt about what to do.

Bronchial Congestion – see Bronchitis

Bruises and Bumps

A bruise is an injury that causes discoloration to the body, without breaking the skin. Usually injury, blood disorders or infections cause these ruptured blood vessels to appear near the surface of the skin or in muscles.

To help reduce bruising to an area, first apply ice wrapped in a cloth or package of frozen vegetables to the traumatized area. Tea tree oil helps reduce inflammation and speeds up the healing process.

Caution   If the damaged area is near the eye do not get tea tree oil in or too close to the eye.

Recommendations

Apply this soothing and healing lotion directly or with a compress. Mix 2 tbsp (1 oz, 30 ml) of distilled witch hazel (Hamamelis water) and 15-20 drops of tea tree oil. Shake lotion vigorously before applying to skin. Apply to the affected area. After applying the lotion cover the area with a moist soft cloth. Keep area moist until relieved.

Apply a cold compress, pad of wet folded cloth to the skin. An easy compress is made by dipping a face cloth or soft fabric such as flannel, into a bowl of cold water. After this, gently dab or massage 1-3 drops of pure tea tree oil onto the affected area.

Bunions

A bunion is an inflamed swelling at the base of the big toe, which can become hardened over time, causing pain. The swelling of the second synovial joint bursa produces displacement and enlargement of the big toe. Eventually it may lap over the second toe.

This hard swollen spot on the foot is an indication of improperly poorly fitted shoes. Children can develop bunions as well as adults. A chiropractor, podiatrist or properly trained foot specialist can fit you or your child in custom made orthodics, which will alleviate some of the discomfort. Well fitted shoes are very important.

In young children, if detected early enough, orthodics can help prevent the leg bones from forming badly and creating the conditions which foster bunions.

Recommendations

Apply pure tea tree oil to the affected joint whenever discomfort exists.

Soak the foot in a bowl of warm water to which you added 4-6 drops of pure tea tree oil.

Soak the foot in a water soluble blend of 1 oz (2 tbsp, 30 ml) of glycerin and 15-25 drops of pure tea tree oil. Shake the mixture vigorously then stir it into the warm water. If you wish, you may add 1 oz (2 tbsp, 30 ml) of Epson salts to the warm water.

Burns

Burns can be caused by heat, light or power through sources such as fire, acids, electricity, sunshine, etcetera. For example a sunburn is an inflammation of the skin from excessive exposure to ultraviolet rays. The usual sources are the sun's rays or a sunlamp. The severity of a burn is explained as follows:

First-degree burn	reddens the skin
Second-degree burn	reddens the skin plus some water blisters form.
Third-degree burn	Contact or see your doctor immediately.

Third degree burns causes lower cell damage, penetrating into muscle and deep tissue, which results in fluid release and may cause breaks in the skin which are where bacteria and infections can enter. The extent of the damage to nerves, lymphatic vessels and deep blood vessels should be assessed by your doctor as soon as possible. If immediate medical attention is not available, follow the recommendations below and then cover the area with a sterile bandage.

Recommendations

Immediately flush the burn with cold water or apply ice wrapped in a face cloth or a frozen package of vegetables to the area, until it is cooled down. Then apply pure tea tree oil to the burn and surrounding area. It can provide quick if not instant relief. In addition its helps prevent the occurrence of infection to the burned area.

If you cannot first cool down the fresh burn with an application of ice or cold, use pure tea tree oil on it immediately.

In most cases a 15% solution of tea tree oil is as effective as a full-strength tea tree oil solution. To burns over larger surface areas, use an atomizer or spray mister with a 15% dilution of tea tree oil in distilled water, aloe vera juice or add your premixed water soluble vegetable glycerin mixture to the distilled water or aloe vera juice.

Do not spray the mister directly onto the burn if the area is very tender. Direct the mist spray above the burn, so it will gently drift down and cover the affected area. Shake the mixture vigorously before using.

To make a 15% tea tree oil water soluble glycerin solution for the skin, mix 30 drops of pure tea tree oil with 1 tsp (1/6 oz, 5 ml) of glycerin and 1 tsp (1/6 oz, 5 ml) aloe vera gel or juice or distilled water or any combination of these adding up to a volume of 2 tsp (1/3 oz, 10 ml). For larger amounts of water soluble glycerin mixtures, the ratio is 1 part tea tree oil to 6 parts of other base liquids or base liquid combinations.

Note   Tea tree oil is about 6 to 7 times more powerful then aloe vera. In combination these two very effectively help manage burns. They are soothing, promote healing, and help prevent secondary infections.

Apply this mixture. The alcohol may cause discomfort or pain to the burn. Mix 1 tbsp (1/2 oz, 15 ml) of isopropyl alcohol and 2 tbsp (1 oz, 30 ml) of pure tea tree oil. Shake vigorously. Let bottle rest on a flat surface for a couple of minutes. If tea tree oil floats to the surface, add more alcohol and shake again, until oil is evenly dispersed in the mixture. Store it in a glass bottle and cool place. This quantity will last for quite a while.

Bursitis

Bursitis is an inflammation of the bursa, small fluid filled shock absorbing sacs, that causes swelling and painful movement to a joint area, such as in the elbow, hip, knee or shoulder. It is beneficial to limit joint motion and apply moist heat to the area during the healing process. Do not exercise the joint until the swelling and pain is reduced. If the pain does not subside in a few days seek medical help.

Recommendations

Apply a compress, pad of wet or medicated folded cloth to the skin. It may be hot or cold.

An easy disinfectant compress is made by dipping a face cloth or soft fabric such as flannel, into a bowl of either steaming hot or ice cold water, that you added 3-6 drops of tea tree oil to.

Apply a poultice to a sore part of the body. To make a poultice stir in 3-6 drops of tea tree oil in a kaolin or clay base. Make sure to mix it well.

Callouses – see Corns

A callous is the hardening and thickening of normal skin caused by friction. Usually caused by repeated pressure to an area, such as feet and hands.

Recommendations

Make sure your shoes are well fitted and softer. Aim to eliminate unnecessary pressure to the affected area. Arch inserts and foam rubber protective bandages may help.

Apply a hot compress, pad of folded cloth soaked in 6 to 10 drops of tea tree oil, to the skin.

Apply a poultice, a hot soft moist mass to calluses. To make a poultice stir in 3-6 drops of tea tree oil in a kaolin or clay base. Make sure to mix it well.

In treating callouses apply pure tea tree oil using a cotton swab or the tip of your finger, directly onto the callous and surrounding area. Then cover the area with an adhesive bandage or band aid. Repeat this on a daily basis until you see results. It may take several weeks or months before the callous is effectively dealt with. Be patient.

Soak your foot in a shallow hot water bath twice a day, for 5-10 minutes. Use this blend in the water: add a blend of 10-20 drops of pure tea tree oil in 1 tbsp (1/2 oz, 15 ml) of a base oil such as avocado, apricot kernel, jojoba, grapeseed, olive or sweet almond oil.

Massage a blend of 8-10 drops of pure tea tree oil mixed with 1 tbsp (1/2 oz, 15 ml) of a carrier base oil such as avocado, apricot kernel, jojoba, grapeseed, olive or sweet almond oil, directly onto the callous. Do two or more times a day.

Canker Sores (Oral) – see Mouth Ulcers

A canker sore is an ulcer-like sore in the mouth, that forms on the inside of the cheeks and gums.

Recommendations

At the first sign of the sore, put a drop of pure tea tree oil on your finger and apply it to the canker sore. Repeat every 4 to 5 hours.

When brushing your teeth, use a commercially prepared tea tree oil toothpaste or put a drop of pure tree tea oil on your regular brand of toothpaste. A good electric tooth brush, gently applied to the gums, tongue and cheeks as well as the teeth, will reduce your mouth's bacterial count.

Gargle with a mouthwash to which you add a couple drops of tea tree oil. Most mouthwashes contain alcohol, add 6-10 drops of tea tree oil to it. The higher the alcohol content the easier the oil will dissolve and stay evenly dispersed in it.

Candida Albicans – see Balantitis, Diaper Rash, Genitourinary
infections, Leucorrhoea/Pruritis,
Mouth and Gum Infection,
Thrush, Vaginal Infection.

Candida infection is also know as moniliasis or candidiasis, which can show itself in many forms. Candida albicans causes a yeast-like fungal infection. It thrives in the warm moist parts of the body such as the mouth (candidiasis), penis (balanitis), vagina (thrush), beneath the breasts and between folds of the buttock (diaper rash). Each condition manifests itself in a slightly different way. Follow the recommendations for each particular condition. It is important to deal with the underlying causes to prevent the recurrence of this yeast-like fungal infection. In chronic cases consult with your health care practitioner.

Professor P. Belaiche at the University of Paris, Phytotherapy Department did a series of studies with tea tree oil. He reported the results in *Phytotherapy*,[11] 1985. One study involved 28 women, with the vaginal infection thrush (Candida albicans). For 30 days vaginal capsules infused with tea tree oil were inserted every evening. The results were twenty-one women were completely healed. Seven women were clinically healed yet not biologically cured.

Carbuncles

Carbuncles is a collective mass of boils caused by the *Staphylococcus aureus*. Characterized by a painful node, covered with tight red skin that later thins and discharges pus.

Commonly found on buttocks, upper back and nape of the neck. Extensive sloughing of the skin occurs when it is healing.

Recommendations

Keep the area clean. Apply pure tea tree oil to the site of the infection, 3-4 times a day.

Soak in a bath. Add 8-12 drops (for children 5 drops) of pure tea tree oil to the water when you are filling up the bath tub. Stir the water once the tub is full. Soak for 10-20 minutes. The penetrating, pain-killing (analgesic) and disinfectant properties of tea tree oil increases the benefits of the bath.

Add half of this 15% tea tree oil water soluble glycerin mixture to the bath water. To make a 15% solution, mix 30 drops of pure tea tree oil with 1 tsp (1/6 oz, 5 ml) of glycerin and 1 tsp (1/6 oz, 5 ml) aloe vera juice or gel. You can use just glycerin in the base, in which case you use 2 tsp (1/3 oz, 10 ml) of glycerin. For larger amounts of water soluble glycerin mixtures, the ratio is 1 part of tea tree oil to 6 parts of other base liquids.

Carpal Tunnel Syndrome

Carpal Tunnel Syndrome is caused by repetitive motions of the wrist. Usually it is associated with constant work at a computer keyboard. When the tendons crowded next to the nerves in the carpal tunnel of the wrist, become overworked, it causes inflammation and swelling. The median nerve gets squeezed as the tendons swell.

Recommendations

Prevention is the best way to deal with this. Through out the day stretch your hands and wrists giving them a time out. Exercise them before you start typing or doing any repetitive tasks, by doing warm up stretches with your hands and wrists for 10 to 15 minutes.

Massage wrists with a blend of 6-8 drops of pure tea tree oil and 1 tbsp (1/2 oz, 15 ml) of a light vegetable oil such as avocado, apricot kernel, jojoba, grapeseed, olive or sweet almond oil. Mix thoroughly before each use. Store in a small container you can carry with you and use each day. Repeat as needed throughout the day. The healing, penetrating and analgesic properties of tea tree oil, combined with the benefits of massage and nourishing your skin with this mix, are very therapeutic for sufferers of this problem.

Chapped Lips

Chapped lips happen as a result of exposure of the mucous membranes of the lips to wind and cold.

Recommendation

Apply a protective coating before being exposed to windy and cold conditions or if lips are already chapped use this blend. Add 1-3 drops of pure tea tree oil to 1 tbsp (1/2 oz, 15 ml) of white petroleum jelly or a light vegetable oil such as avocado, apricot kernel, jojoba, grapeseed, olive or sweet almond oil. Mix thoroughly with a toothpick. Store in a small container you can carry with you. This amount will last for a while. Dip your finger in the blend and cover your lips with it. If lips are chapped, then apply every 20-30 minutes, they will be restored to normal within 2-12 hours.

Chickenpox – same treatment used for Shingles or Zona

Chickenpox is an acute, highly contagious viral disease, especially during childhood. It is caused by the *Herpes zoster* virus, the same one responsible for shingles. It is characterized by skin eruptions of itchy spots, that blister, then turn to crusts.

Tea tree oil's anti-viral, analgesic (pain-killing), diaphoretic (sweat promoting) and immune system stimulating properties, make it a powerful and very effective tool to help deal with chickenpox. The additional benefits of soothing itches and its therapeutic healing properties, helps to prevent scarring and infection due to scratching.

In a 1986 issue of *Aromatherapy Quarterly*,[19, 20] a severe case of chickenpox in an 11 month old baby was reported. Using 2 drops of pure tea tree oil and 1 drop of essential oil of German chamomile in the bath water, they saw noticeable improvement in the babies condition within an hour. After a couple more baths, the baby slept soundly. By morning *'most the blisters were*

50% smaller, and all those that erupted from this time onwards remained small. They continued bathing the baby, until all the scabs fell off.'

In teenagers and adults chickenpox is much more dangerous, as it causes high fever and can be very painful.

Recommendations

Use vaporizers, to which you add 5 drops of pure tea tree oil to the water, for the duration of the chickenpox. Remember to refresh the water reservoir with tea tree oil. If you do not have a vaporizer, add 5 drops of pure tea tree oil to 2 cups (16 oz, 473 ml) of boiling water to freshen and add healing properties to the air.

Apply this protective, soothing, healing and drying lotion. To 2 tbsp (1 oz, 30 ml) of calamine lotion add 15-20 drops (5 drops for children) of pure tea tree oil. Shake lotion vigorously before applying to skin. Apply 3-4 times daily.

Apply this soothing and healing lotion. Mix 4 tbsp (2 oz, 60 ml) of distilled witch hazel (Hamamelis water) and 5-8 drops of tea tree oil. Shake lotion vigorously before applying to skin. Apply repeatedly to the affected area using a gauze cloth or cotton ball.

Note   This is not recommended for young babies. Consult your doctor.

To bath water add 8-10 drops (for children 2-4 drops, and they must be closely supervised, to make sure they do not get it in their eyes or mouth) of pure tea tree oil to an anti-itch oatmeal (colloidal oatmeal) bath available from drug stores and pharmacies. 'Aveena' is a colloidal oatmeal product. Save money by grinding up raw oatmeal into a fine powder and using it in the bath water.

Here is what adult patients have done: Used calamine lotion... soaked in anti-itch oatmeal suspension... dabbed pure tea tree oil on their facial pox spots a few times a day... used other essential oils, in combination with tea tree oil. To find various formulae and which essential oils to use, check with your health food store or supplier of pure essential oils. Aromatherapy books have suitable suggestions.

Note   Teenagers and adults should consult with their health care
          provider at the earliest sign of chickenpox.

Chiggers

Chiggers are the tiny red larva of certain mites, whose bite
causes severe itching. They live mainly in Midwestern and
Southern states. To feed the larva bore into skin pores and follicles, causing itching and a rash.

Recommendations

Massage pure tea tree oil into the sites of the bites, once in
the morning and once at night.

Soak in a warm bath. Add 8-12 drops of pure tea tree oil to
the warm water when you are filling up the bath tub. Stir the
water once the tub is full. Soak for 10-20 minutes. The penetrating, anti-itching and pain-killing (analgesic) properties of tea
tree oil increase the benefits of the bath.

To bath water add 8-10 drops (for children 2-4 drops, and
they must be closely supervised, to make sure they do not get it
in their eyes or mouth) of pure tea tree oil to an anti-itch oatmeal
(colloidal oatmeal) bath available from drug stores and pharmacies. 'Aveena' is a colloidal oatmeal product. Save money by
grinding up raw oatmeal into a fine powder and using it in the
bath water. Ask your health care practitioner if an oatmeal
suspension is suitable for you.

Preventative: Spray a mist of this solution on your pant leg
bottoms and socks: 8-10 drops of tea tree oil to 1 cup (8 oz, 237
ml) of water. Shake the spray mister vigorously before each
application.

Chilblains

Chilblains is a painful swelling or sore, especially on the
fingers or toes, caused by exposure to the cold or poor circulation. They are generally small, painful reddish-blue swellings,
which can be itchy. Nutritional deficiencies may contribute to
the problem. Preventative measures include exercise and warm
clothing.

Recommendations

Apply pure tea tree oil to the chilblain.

Massage the affected area(s) to improve blood circulation. Mix 6-9 drops of pure tea tree oil with 1 tbsp (1/2 oz, 15 ml) of a light vegetable base carrier oil such as avocado, jojoba, grapeseed, olive, sweet almond oil, etcetera. Shake or mix the contents vigorously before each application. A little will go a long way. Apply to the affected area 2 to 4 times daily, then reduce to twice daily.

Chronic Fatigue – see Immune System

Clavus – see Corn

Colds – see Coughs, Fever, Flu, Sinusitis, Sore Throat

A cold is a viral infection of the respiratory track. It may cause sneezing, coughing, running nose, congestion, fever, aches and pains, etcetera. On average a cold lasts 7-8 days.

It is important to note that a cold may lead to complications. The young, elderly and chronically ill should seek medical help as soon as possible, if fever gets too high or the condition gets worse.

Tea tree oil can be beneficial by combating the infection, easing the coughing, helping the lungs rid themselves of mucus and reducing the fever. In addition it reinforces the body's immune system and prevents the spread of the infection.

Recommendations

As soon as the condition occurs, start steam inhalation to help prevent the infection from developing any further and to soothe coughing. To a bowl of steaming hot water add 5 drops of pure tea tree oil and inhale for 5 to 10 minutes. If you want to capture more of the steam, drape a towel over your head and the bowl. Make sure the table and bowl are very stable and secure. Be very careful not to spill any of the hot water and burn or scald yourself.

Drink plenty of water and a commercially prepared tea tree oil preparation – either hot or as a refreshing ice cold tea. Hot is better in terms of helping to break up the mucus. Some cold sufferers add 1 drop of pure tea tree oil, to 1 tsp (1/6 oz, 5 ml) of honey and blend it with 2 cups of camomile or other herbal tea. The drink may help stimulate your compromised immune system.

Take a hot bath. Put 8-12 drops (only 5 drops for children) of pure tea tree oil in the water, when filling the bath tub. Stir water to disperse the oil. This encourages your body to sweat, which is its natural reaction to fever. The effect is similar to doing steam inhalation. If feverish, especially if the bodies temperature is high, use cool water in the bath.

Massage the back, chest and throat with a blend of 2.5% tea tree oil. As a base use 1 tsp (1/6 oz, 5 ml) of a light oil such as avocado, apricot kernel, jojoba, grapeseed, olive or sweet almond oil. If you plan to frequently massage the back, chest and throat use 1 tbsp (1/2 oz, 15 ml) of light vegetable oil and 9 drops of tea tree oil.

Massage upper back and chest with a blend of 2.5% pure tea tree oil (9 drops) and 1 tbsp (1/2 oz, 15 ml) Friar's Balsam (Active ingredients: Benzoin, aloe, storax, Tolu balsam. Inactive ingredients: Alcohol). Repeat twice a day. You can use the same mixture in your humidifier. It relieves bronchial congestion and has numerous other benefits.

Inhalation using a vaporizer in your bedroom at night is very beneficial. Put 5 drops of pure tea tree oil in your vaporizer at home. Boost the benefits by adding 2-3 drops of pure tea tree oil to 1 tsp (1/6 oz, 5 ml) of eucalyptus oil and put this mixture in the vaporizer or add the tea tree oil and eucalyptus oil mixture to 2 cups (16 oz, 473 ml) of boiling water to freshen and add healing benefits to the air.

On a handkerchief or kleenex tissue put a few drops of tea tree oil for inhalation during the day. At night put a drop on your pillow, just below your nose.

Wash your hands thoroughly using tea tree oil soap. Triclosan is the active ingredient which laboratory testing shows destroys harmful bacteria like Strep., E. coli, Salmonella, Staph and viruses. This helps prevent the transmission of disease causing agents.

Note Consult your family health care provider, if condition worsens, or you are in doubt about what to do.

Cold Sores (Herpes Simplex 1)

Cold sores are a viral infection, brought on by the herpes simplex virus 1, causing inflammation to the skin, usually the lips, mouth and face. It is characterized by small blisters. Herpes simplex 1 is highly infectious and can spread to other parts of the body.

In 1991, a clinical study by Mayo and Shemesh, revealed the effectiveness of tea tree oil, for the treatment of this difficult and recurring problem.

Cold sores may occur with a fever, infection or cold, during menstruation, under stress, exposure to sun and wind or when your immune system is depressed. After exposure, it may take 3 to 10 days for them to appear and they can last up to 3 weeks.

Recommendations

As soon as sore spots develop, soak a cotton swab in tea tree oil and dab onto the spot. Early treatment prevents the cold sores from developing any further. Repeat frequently until the condition disappears. It may take several days.

In the initial stages before the blisters break open, instead of pure tea tree oil, you can use a grain alcohol based solution. Add 6 drops of pure tea tree oil to 1 tsp (1/6 oz, 5 ml) of a grain alcohol such as vodka. Massage it into the area affected.

Congestion – see Coughs

Coral Cuts – see Cuts

Coral cuts are often irregular and jagged deep cuts that make a perfect breeding ground and harbor for bacteria. It is important to remove any coral and sand particles from the wound. Wash the cuts in pure water then disinfect it with a few drops of pure tea tree oil. When wounds cut through the skin and into muscle, it is important to have them sutured. This speeds up healing and reduces the chances of secondary infection. Check daily for swelling or redness, indications of infection. Apply a few drops of pure tea tree oil to the gauze bandage used to cover the suture and wound.

Additional Recommendation

Apply this mixture. The alcohol in it may cause discomfort or pain to the cut. Mix 1 tbsp (1/2 oz, 15 ml) of isopropyl alcohol and 2 tbsp (1 oz, 30 ml) of pure tea tree oil. Shake vigorously. Let bottle rest on a flat surface for a couple of minutes. If tea tree oil floats to the surface add more alcohol and shake again until oil is evenly dispersed in the mixture. Store it in a glass bottle and cool place. This quantity will last for quite a while and may be used as a disinfectant.

Corns

A corn, also called a clavus, is an area of thickened hard skin between or on the toes. Sometimes it forms an inverted pyramid, which causes pressure in deeper layers of skin, resulting in pain. It is the result of ill fitted shoes causing pressure and friction over the bony parts of the foot, such as toe joints and ball of the foot. A clinical study by Dr. Walker,[9] indicated a significant degree of success using tea tree oil to treat corns and other problems related to health conditions of feet.

Recommendations

In treating corns apply pure tea tree oil, using a cotton swab or the tip of your finger, directly on the corn and surrounding area. Then cover the area with an adhesive bandage or band aid. Repeat this on a daily basis until you see results. It may take several weeks or months before the corn is effectively dealt with. Be patient.

Soak your foot in a shallow hot water bath twice a day. Use this blend in the water: blend 10-20 drops of pure tea tree oil with 1 tbsp (1/2 oz, 15 ml) of a base oil such as avocado, apricot kernel, jojoba, grapeseed, olive or sweet almond oil. Once the corn is softened enough you should be able to easily remove it with tweezers. Apply a drop of pure tea tree oil to the exposed skin and cover with a small bandage.

Massage a blend of 8-10 drops of pure tea tree oil mixed with 1 tbsp (1/2 oz, 15 ml) of a base oil such as avocado, apricot kernel, jojoba, grapeseed, olive or sweet almond oil, directly on the corn. Do two or more times a day. Once the corn is softened enough, you should be able to easily remove it with tweezers. Apply a drop of pure tea tree oil to the exposed skin and cover with a small bandage.

Coughs

Coughing is a natural reflex whose purpose is to clear a blockage or irritation from the respiratory tract. Coughs are either dry or cause the discharge of mucus, especially in the case of bronchitis, flu or colds. The lungs can become congested with mucous. Coughing helps clear them.

The acute cough is temporary and short term in nature usually indicating a blockage or irritation in the respiratory tract.

The chronic cough is long-term and warrants seeking medical help.

The following conditions may aggravate a cough: Smoking, secondhand smoke, air pollution, a damp climate, improper diet – such as too many dairy products and poor nutrition.

The young, elderly and chronically ill should seek medical help as soon as possible, if the condition gets worse.

Tea tree oil can be of benefit due to its strong anti-viral, bactericidal, expectorant and balsamic properties. If infection or inflammation is present, it is a very valuable remedy to ease the coughing. In addition it reinforces the body's immune system and prevents the spread of the infection.

Recommendations

As soon as the condition occurs, start steam inhalation to soothe coughing and lessen congestion. To a bowl of steaming hot water add 5 drops of pure tea tree oil and inhale for 5 to 10 minutes. If you want to capture more of the steam, drape a towel over your head and the bowl. Make sure the table and bowl are very stable and secure. Be very careful not to spill any of the hot water and burn or scald yourself. Repeat twice daily.

Drink plenty of water and a tea tree oil herbal tea – either hot or as a refreshing ice cold tea. A long time tea tree oil user finds this helps them. They add a drop of pure tea tree oil to a teaspoon of honey and to 2 cups of chamomile or other soothing herbal tea. They find hot is better in terms of breaking up the mucus. The drink may help stimulate your compromised immune system. We suggest you buy a commercially prepared tea tree oil tea.

Take a bath. Put 8-12 drops (5 or less drops for children) of pure tea tree oil into the bath water. This encourages your body to sweat, which is its natural reaction to fever. The effect is similar to doing steam inhalation. If feverish, especially if the bodies temperature is high, use cool water in the bath – but it will not have the same benefits of steam inhalation.

Massage the back, chest and throat with a blend of 2.5% pure tea tree oil. Add 3 drops of tea tree oil to a base of 1 tsp (1/6 oz, 5 ml) of a light oil such as avocado, apricot kernel, jojoba, grape-seed, olive or sweet almond oil. If you plan to frequently massage the back, chest and throat use 2 tbsp (1 oz, 30 ml) of the light vegetable oil and 18 drops of pure tea tree oil. Repeat up to 4 times daily.

Massage upper back and chest with a blend of 2.5% pure tea tree oil (9 drops) and 1 tbsp (1/2 oz, 15 ml) Friar's Balsam (Active ingredients: Benzoin, aloe, storax, Tolu balsam. Inactive ingredients: Alcohol). Repeat twice a day. You can use the same mixture in your humidifier. It relieves bronchial congestion and has numerous other benefits.

Massage a few drops of pure tea tree oil into the chest and back.

Inhalation using a vaporizer is very beneficial. Add 5 drops of pure tea tree oil to the water in your vaporizer at home. Boost the benefits by adding 2-3 drops of pure tea tree oil to 1 tsp (1/6 oz, 5 ml) of eucalyptus oil and put this mixture in the vaporizer or add the tea tree oil and eucalyptus oil mixture to 2 cups (16 oz, 473 ml) of boiling water to freshen and add healing proper-ties to the air. It is very effective when sleeping.

On a handkerchief or facial tissue put a few drops of pure tea tree oil for inhalation throughout the day.

At night, sprinkle a few drops of pure tea tree oil onto your pillow.

Note   Consult your family health care provider, if condition worsens, or you are in doubt about what to do.

Crabs – see Head Lice

Crabs are a lice infestation of the pubic hairs.

Cradle Cap

Cradle cap is a form of dermatitis newborn and very young babies exhibit. This unsightly scalp condition is thick yellowish crust lesions which develop on the scalp, face and sometimes extend to a scaling behind the ears.

Recommendations

Prepare a fresh mixture of 4-5 drops of tea tree oil blended with 1 tsp (1/6 oz, 5 ml) of cold pressed virgin olive oil. Put the mixture in your hand and let it warm to your body temperature before gently applying it to the babies scalp. Do not get any into the babies eyes. Leave it for 5-8 minutes before applying a tea tree oil shampoo to wash it out. A slightly oily residue may be left after treatment. Next, rinse the scalp again making sure to protect the babies eyes. Initially repeat this daily until the condition improves. Once the problem is resolved a good preventative measure is using tea tree oil shampoo to wash the babies scalp.

Tip   To make a tea tree oil shampoo, add 5-12 drops of pure tea tree oil into the bottle of shampoo. Label bottle – *Tea Tree Added*. Shake bottle vigorously each time before you use it.

Cramps

Cramps are a sudden painful involuntary contraction of muscles during or after strenuous activity or strain or chills caused due to low calcium and low oxygen levels in that muscle.

After a meal, wait an hour before exercising. Before exercising do warm up and stretching exercises to prevent cramps. Hormonal changes, such as menstruation can also cause cramps. Proper nutrition or supplementation may alleviate or prevent hormonal imbalances from causing the problem in the future. A warm bath and massage can alleviate the pain greatly.

Recommendations

Soak in a warm bath. Add 8-12 drops of pure tea tree oil to the warm water when you are filling up the bath tub. Once the tub is full, stir the water. Soak for 10-20 minutes. The penetrating and pain-killing (analgesic) properties of tea tree oil increases the benefits of the bath.

Muscular spasms or very tight areas can be relieved by massaging a few drops of pure tee tree oil into the affected area. You can also add a few drops of pure tea tree oil to a warm compress and apply it to the area.

Massage the affected muscular aches and pains areas with this massage oil: Mix 9 drops of pure tea tree oil in 1 tbsp (1/2 oz, 15 ml) of a light base oil such as jojoba, grapeseed or sweet almond oil. Mix thoroughly. Repeat as often as needed.

Caution   Pregnant or lactating women should consult with a health care practitioner, before using tea tree oil.

Cuticles – see Nails (Infected)

Cuticles are the hardened layer of outside skin, at the base and sides of a fingernail.

Cuts

A cut is an injury to the tissue and should be treated as soon as possible after injury. Early treatment with tea tree oil prevents infection, and at the same time does not cause damage to the healthy tissue surrounding the cut. It is an excellent antiseptic and has wound healing properties. In addition to this it does not sting the raw exposed skin.

In the 1930's E. Humphrey reported in an article in the *Medical Journal of Australia*, that tea tree oil worked better as a germicide, in the presence of dirt or pus.

Recommendations

Clean and wash affected area with a soft cloth and warm water. Apply a few drops of pure tea tree oil and a bandage if needed. Repeat several times a day until the skin has healed.

For minor cuts mix 1-2 drops of pure tea tree oil with some honey and apply to the affected area. Cover with a Band Aid or gauze. Change dressing daily and repeat as needed.

Apply this mixture. The alcohol in it may cause discomfort or pain. Mix 1 tbsp (1/2 oz, 15 ml) of grain alcohol and 2 tbsp (1 oz, 30 ml) of pure tea tree oil. Shake vigorously. Let bottle rest on a flat surface for a couple of minutes. If tea tree oil floats to the surface add more alcohol and shake again until the oil is evenly dispersed in it. Store it in a glass bottle and a cool place. This quantity will last for quite a while and has many additional uses, such as a disinfectant.

Cracked Dry Skin – see Frostbite, Psoriasis, Eczema, Fungal Infections, Viral Skin Infections

Dry cracked skin on the hands and feet is a common problem in cold climate winter conditions. Severe cases are painful especially for those suffering with psoriasis, frostbite or similar skin conditions. It is important to moisturize and protect the skin from infection and further damage.

Note   Cracked dry skin on the foot can be an indication of a viral or fungal infection. Check with your health care practitioner for the diagnosis and try the appropriate tea tree oil treatments for those conditions listed in this book.

Recommendations

Apply a 15% tea tree oil water soluble glycerin mixture to the skin. To make this 15% solution mix 30 drops of pure tea tree oil with 1 tsp (1/6 oz, 5 ml) of glycerin and 1 tsp (1/6 oz, 5 ml) aloe vera juice or gel. You can use just glycerin in the base, in which case you use 2 tsp (1/3 oz, 10 ml). For larger amounts of water soluble glycerin mixtures, the ratio is approximately 1 part of tea tree oil to 6 parts of other base liquids.

Apply a tea tree and wheat germ oil mixture. Mix 3 drops of tea tree oil with 1 tsp (1/6 oz, 5 ml) of wheat germ oil or a good moisturizing cream. Massage into the affected area once in the morning, at lunchtime and at night until the condition improves. After improvement, as preventative measure, apply the tea tree moisturizing mixture daily.

Cystitis – see Urethritis

Cystitis is a bladder infection caused by bacteria. It is more common in women than men.

Urethritis a bacterial infection of the urethra which usually precedes an attack of cystitis. A sign of cystitis is the need to urinate frequently, accompanied with a painful burning sensation while urinating and sometimes feeling feverish. The urine may look cloudy.

Proper hygiene is an important preventative measure. Women should wipe themselves, with a downward stroke, starting from the urethra toward the anus. Men should wash frequently, making sure to thoroughly clean the area surrounding and under the foreskin.

In the 1980's, Dr. P. Belaiche[11] reported successfully treating chronic cystitis using tea tree oil. Of particular note was how effective he found Melaleuca alternifolia tea tree oil in treating chronic colibacilli cystitis. Very little irritation to the mucous membrane, absence of toxicity and high germicidal properties make this an excellent antiseptic in aromatherapy applications.

Caution   Any internal application of pure or diluted mixtures of tea tree oil, should be supervised by your health care practitioner. See your doctor immediately if there is pus or blood in the urine or the symptoms do not improve within a few days.

Recommendations

Flush your system by drinking distilled water. Wear loose fitting clothes and cotton underwear in addition to any one or combination of the following:

Swab the opening of the urethra each time after urination with a cotton ball soaked in a tea tree oil solution with distilled or cold boiled water. Use a clean glass container with a good sealing top. To 1 cup (8 oz, 237 ml) of distilled or cold boiled water add 5 drops of tea tree oil. Shake vigorously each time before using, since the oil does not stay evenly suspended in water solutions.

Drink a commercially prepared tea tree oil tea frequently throughout the day.

To bath water add 8-12 drops of pure tea tree oil. Mix it in thoroughly. Soak for 5-10 minutes. Frequent bathing with tea tree oil as a general disinfectant is a good preventative measure.

Apply a massage oil gently to the lower back and abdomen. Mix 3 drops of pure tea tree oil in 1 tsp (5 ml) of a light base oil such as jojoba, grapeseed or sweet almond oil. Mix thoroughly. Repeat 2 or more times daily.

Dandruff

Dandruff is a condition affecting the scalp. Overactive sebaceous gland secretions in the scalp cause scales to form, which may itch and burn.

It may be caused by poor diet, inadequate stimulation of the scalp, poor blood circulation, pityrosporum ovale yeast which lives on the scalp, Candida albicans, trichoplyton spp fungi, stress or chemical hair preparations.

Tea tree oil can clear up the problem and an added bonus is it improves the health of your hair.

Recommendations

Blend 30 drops of pure tea tree oil with 1/4 cup (2 oz, 60 ml) of warmed coconut or jojoba oil. Massage into your scalp. If possible, wrap warm towels around your head. To remove the massage oil, you must first work in a 2-3% tea tree oil shampoo or blend 5 drops of pure tea tree oil with 1 tsp (1/6 oz, 5 ml) of a neutral pH balanced mild shampoo into your hair. Once the shampoo is thoroughly worked in you rinse it with water. The order is very important, since the shampoo helps remove most of the oil from your scalp and hair. Repeat weekly.

On a daily or regular basis use a 2-3% tea tree oil shampoo

or make your own. Add 20 drops (1/5 tsp, 1/30 oz, 1 ml) of tea tree oil for each ounce (2 tbsp, 30 ml) of a neutral pH balanced shampoo. Here's an example for a larger volume: Add 80 drops (4/5 tsp, 4 ml) of tea tree oil to 1/2 cup (4 oz, 118 ml) of shampoo. Shake vigorously before each use.

Note   It is suggested that you vary the brand of shampoo you use for a base, since after extended use of the same shampoo, it becomes less effective as a cleaning agent. When you finish one bottle, switch brands, then switch back to the original brand. This problem is a result of the chemical build ups that occur over time.

In a rush!? A quick method you can use between washes, if needed, is to vigorously massage a few drops of pure tea tree oil into your scalp and hair. This helps unblock the hair follicles.

Dental Plaque

Dental plague is a build up of hardened material around the teeth. It can affect your gums and the general state of your mouth's health if allowed to build up and remain.

In Australia dentists use a tea tree oil mouthwash to sterilize cavities before filling. Frequent users of tea tree oil toothpaste have indicated that plaque is no longer a problem for them. One said, "My dental hygienist asked me if I had my teeth recently cleaned since the last time I had been there a year ago." "No. Why?" I asked her. "There's hardly any plaque in your mouth."

According to an Australian official, Colgate-Palmolive tested a tea tree oil toothpaste. Since it could not secure a sufficient quantity of pure tea tree oil to satisfy the American market, it discontinued the test and decided not to produce it for commercial purposes.

Using the following methods can help soften plaque and reduce its formation.

Brush frequently or at least twice a day using a tea tree oil toothpaste, or add a drop of tea tree oil to your regular toothpaste before brushing.

Create your own tea tree toothpaste. Blend in 12-15 drops with 1 tbsp (1/2 oz, 15 ml) of your favorite toothpaste. To enhance the benefits of tea tree oil toothpaste, a good electric toothbrush is definitely worth investing in.

Rinse and hold a tea tree oil mouthwash in your mouth for 1 minute. You can create your own by adding 6-8 drops of tea tree oil for each ounce of the mouthwash. Most mouthwashes contain alcohol, which tea tree oil dissolves in. The more alcohol content a mouthwash contains, the easier the oil will dissolve and stay evenly dispersed in it. Shake the bottle each time before gargling. Beneficial for the gums which can be damaged by excessive plaque build up.

If you do not have or use mouthwash you can rinse the mouth at least twice daily with a solution of 7-8 drops of pure tea tree oil, mixed well in a glass of 8 oz of warm water. Rinse every morning and evening after brushing the teeth.

Dermatitis – see Cracked Dry Skin, Cradle Cap,
                    Eczema, Psoriasis.

Dermatitis is an inflammation of the skin. Characteristics may include flaky skin, redness, itchiness and rashes resulting in blisters, sores and scabs.

The following is a list of possible causes: detergents, soaps, cosmetics, pollution, sunlight, hot weather, heredity, allergies to food products like milk and wheat. The actual cause may be hard to find since the reaction may take time to appear. Mental and emotional stress tends to aggravate or trigger attacks.

Recommendations

Identify and remove the cause of the problem. Deal with mental and emotional stresses by learning relaxation or meditation techniques.

Massage pure tea tree oil into the affected area.

For larger areas make a water-based lotion. Add 30 drops of tea tree oil to 1/2 cup (4 oz, 118 ml) of distilled water. Shake vigorously before each application. Apply twice daily to the affected area.

Apply this soothing and healing lotion. Mix 2 tbsp (1 oz, 30 ml) of distilled witch hazel (Hamamelis water) and 15-20 drops of tea tree oil. Shake lotion vigorously then apply to the affected area.

Wash with a tea tree oil soap.

To bath water add 8-12 drops of pure tea tree oil. Mix it in thoroughly.

To bath water add a water soluble glycerin base mixture. In the container first put 2 oz (4 tbsp, 60 ml) of vegetable glycerin add 1 oz (2 tbsp, 30 ml) of full-strength tea tree oil and 1 oz (2 tbsp, 30 ml) of water. Tightly seal the container. Finally shake the mixture vigorously then add to bath water.

Moisturize your skin by massaging a tea tree oil moisturizer in the affected areas. If you are using a moisturizer already, add a few drops of pure tea tree oil to it, to increase its effectiveness.

Massage with this healing combinations of oils. They are particularly effective base oils for eczema and psoriasis. Add 15-18 drops of pure tea tree oil to 1/8 cup (1 oz, 2 tbsp, 30 ml) of a cold pressed light vegetable carrier oil such as sweet almond or corn oil. For up to 10% of the base carrier oil's volume you can use avocado pear, borage, carrot, evening primrose, jojoba, sesame or wheat germ oils. Shake or mix the contents well before each application. A little will go a long way. Apply where and as needed.

Dhobi Itch – see Tinea

Dhobi itch is a fungal infection. It is caused by *Tinea cruris,* generally affecting men in hot climates and during the summer. Inflamed pimples break out on the inside part of the upper thigh, mass together to make a red, scaly and itchy patch with a clearly defined border. This condition can be very irritating and uncomfortable.

Recommendation

Wear all natural clothing that allows the skin to breathe. Cotton shorts and cotton underwear are helpful. When washing clothes add a few drops of pure tea tree oil to the wash water.

Wash the location of the infection and make sure to dry it thoroughly. Then apply pure tea tree oil 2-3 times a day.

Diaper Rash

Diaper rash can be caused by *Candida albicans*. It thrives in the warm moist parts of the body between folds of the buttock.

Recommendations

Keep baby's bottom dry by leaving their bottom's exposed to the air. According to mothers, breast fed babies do not get as much diaper rash, even after the breast feedings have stopped.

Apply Zinc ointment (Active ingredient: 15% zinc oxide – Inactive ingredients: anhydrous lanolin, cetostearyl alcohol, paraffin, white petroleum) to which you added 1-2 drops of pure tea tree oil. Do not use pure tea tree oil alone, on a baby's bottom. The astringent nature of zinc oxide, combined with the therapeutic properties of tea tree oil are very beneficial to the irritated area. Apply as needed, whenever you change the diapers.

Apply this soothing and healing lotion. Mix 2 tbsp (1 oz, 30 ml) of distilled witch hazel (Hamamelis water) and 2-4 drops of pure tea tree oil. Shake lotion vigorously before applying to skin. Apply to the affected area as needed.

Use a commercially prepared tea tree oil cream. Apply as per directions.

Mothers have said this combination works wonders, when all else fails. Massage this combination onto the diaper rash and surrounding area. Add 2-3 drops of pure tea tree oil to 1 tsp (1/6 oz, 5 ml) of wheat germ oil. Mix thoroughly before each application. Apply as needed.

Diabetic Gangrene

Diabetic gangrene is a complication of diabetes, causing the tissue to die. As the condition progresses, amputation of the effected limb is the traditional course of action allopathic medicine recommends.

In 1936 a life threatening severe case of diabetic gangrene was successfully treated with an aqueous (water) suspension of tea tree oil. It was reported in *The Medical Journal of Australia* and cited by Dr. A. Penfold in his article "Some notes on the

Essential Oil of Melaleuca alternifolia,' in the *Australian Journal of Pharmacy*, March 30, 1937. The following points were noted: wound healing without any suppuration, under this antiseptic treatment there was reorganization of slough and necrosed bone, when dressing the wound there was little irritation, application of other antiseptics was minimized.

A study conducted at the Royal North Shore Hospital, Sydney, Australia, by Dr. Jill Fogerty indicated a major difference on the legs of geriatric and diabetic patients using a hand and body lotion containing 5% pure tea tree oil. Benefits included cracks healing and disappearing and softer skin. This is due to the bactericide and skin salve properties of tea tree oil.

Recommendations

Make a 5% dilution of tea tree oil by mixing it with a non-allergenic cream or lotion. For 1 tbsp (1/2 oz, 15 ml) of base use 15 drops of pure tea tree oil. For 1/4 cup (4 tbsp, 2 oz, 60 ml) use 60 drops of essential tea tree oil. Commercially available tea tree ointments are available. Massage into the affected spot and surrounding area. Frequently, the longer a condition exists, the longer it may take to get results. Try this in consultation with your medical practitioner.

To boost the above to a more potent mixture of 15% tea tree oil, use three times the amount of tea tree oil to the same amount of cream or lotion. For 1 tbsp (1/2 oz, 15 ml) of base use 45 drops of pure tea tree oil. For 1/4 cup (4 tbsp, 2 oz, 60 ml) use 180 drops of essential tea tree oil. According to studies, a 15% solution can be as effective as pure tea tree oil.

Massage pure tea tree oil into the affected area and surrounding tissue for as long as needed.

Share this information with your health care provider to better assist you in the management of this condition.

Dust Mites – see Hives

Earaches – see Ear Infections, Ear Wax

Earaches do not mean that you have an infection or hardened

ear wax. If possible, first determine the cause of the pain. Prevent earaches by covering children's ears in windy or cold weather. When landing in an airplane, to help equalize the pressure differential that can cause an earache you can: Chew gum or suck on a hard candy. Place the open end of styrofoam, plastic or cardboard cups over the ears. Works wonders.

Recommendations

To a 1/4 cup (2 oz, 60 ml) of extra virgin olive oil or other neutral oil, add 5-10 drops of pure tea tree oil. Warm to body temperature. The mixture will not feel cold or warm on the skin. Saturate the end of a piece of twisted and pulled cotton with the mixture and insert it loosely into the outside ear canal. This keeps the oils from running out at night. Do not use pure tea tree oil in sensitive ears, as it can irritate them. Repeat as required.

If a live bug is in the ear then use a drop of pure tea tree oil to kill it. You will then be able to safely and painlessly remove the bug.

Caution   Do not use a cotton tipped piece of cardboard, plastic or wood since it can irritate or pierce the ear drum. Consult with your health care provider if earache persists and to find out the underlying cause of the problem.

Ear Infections

Ear infections are very common in babies and young children. Some youth and adults are prone to them particularly after swimming in polluted or highly chlorinated waters. Ear plugs are recommended for those who catch ear infections due to swimming in harsh water. Care should be used when using tea tree oil for babies and young children.

Recommendation

Add 5-10 drops of warm pure tea tree oil to 1 tbsp (1/2 oz, 15 ml) of warm sweet almond or extra virgin olive oil. For stubborn ear infections a 15% dilution is preferred. You do this by increasing the amount of pure tea tree oil to 30 drops for 1 tbsp (1/2 oz, 15 ml) of sweet almond or extra virgin olive oil. Make sure to thoroughly mix this blend before using it in the ear. Trickle a small amount into the child's or adult's ear. Use as needed.

Ear wax

Ear wax is naturally produced to trap dust and protect your ears from it. The wax moves from the ear canal to the ear opening then is bathed away when you wash around your ears. Sometimes the wax gets jammed up. This creates an uncomfortable sometimes itchy condition. In addition the ear is more susceptible to infection.

Recommendation

Try this for hardened or excessive earwax build up. Apply 1 drop of pure tea tree oil to a small piece of cotton which has been twisted and pulled to a point. Gently insert the soaked cotton piece into the ear overnight. The next day, remove the cotton piece and irrigate the ear using a rubber ear syringe filled with water heated to your body temperature. (You can buy a rubber ear syringe at any drug store.) The water should not feel warm or cold to the touch. Place the rubber ear syringe on the side of the ear canal just inside the opening. Gently squeeze a stream of water into the canal, leaving space for the water to carry the dislodged and melted wax out of the ear. Repeated applications may be required.

Caution　　Do not use a cotton swab tipped piece of cardboard, plastic or wood since it can irritate or pierce the ear drum. Consult with your health care provider if the wax build up is too hard or too large.

Eczema – see Dermatitis

Eczema is a skin disorder characterized by inflammation, itching and scaliness. While similar treatments are used for other skin conditions, generally called dermatitis, with eczema it is important to keep the skin dry.

The following is a list of possible causes: detergents, soaps, cosmetics, pollution, sunlight, hot weather, heredity, allergies to food products like milk and wheat. The actual cause may be hard to find, since the reaction may take time to appear. Mental and emotional stress tends to aggravate or trigger attacks.

Recommendations

Keep the skin dry. Identify and remove the cause of the problem. Deal with mental and emotional stresses by learning relaxation or meditation techniques.

Massage pure tea tree oil into the affected area.

For larger areas make a water soluble glycerin based lotion. Add 15 drops of tea tree oil to 1/4 cup (2 oz, 60 ml) of distilled water. Shake vigorously before each application. Apply twice daily to the affected area. A commercially prepared tea tree oil lotion or cream may be used.

Massage with this healing combinations of oils. The base oils are particularly effective for eczema. Add 15-18 drops of pure tea tree oil to 1/8 cup (1 oz, 2 tbsp, 30 ml) of a cold pressed light vegetable carrier oil such as sweet almond or corn oil. For up to 10% of the base carrier oil's volume you can use avocado pear, borage, carrot, evening primrose, jojoba, sesame or wheat germ oils. Shake or mix the contents well before each application. A little will go a long way. Apply as needed.

Moisturize your skin by massaging a tea tree oil moisturizer into the affected areas or blend 2-3 drops of pure tea tree oil with 1 tbsp (1/2 oz, 15 ml) of a non-allergenic moisturizer to increase its effectiveness. Apply to the skin as needed.

Wash with a tea tree oil soap.

Emphysema – see Bronchitis

Emphysema is a condition of the lungs in which the air sacs become distended and lose elasticity.

Fever – see Colds

Fever is an abnormally increased body temperature, which is a vital part of your body's defense mechanism. It strengthens the body's natural defense mechanism and speeds up the body's metabolic rate.

In some, not all cases, it is wise to allow a fever to run its course, which may result in a lot of sweating that eventually subsides. If fever rises to dangerous levels or remains high, seek medical help immediately.

Tea tree oil is a very effective tool in dealing with fevers, since it has such a wide range of actions – anti-viral, bacterial and immune system stimulating properties.

Note   Consult your family health care provider, if fever stays high or rises to a dangerous level.

Recommendations

Use a vaporizer to which you add 3-5 drops of pure tea tree oil to the water in the reservoir. It is important to do this at the fevers onset and during the entire length of the illness.

Control high temperatures by immersing the entire body in tepid bath water. Add 3-12 of pure tea tree oil, depending on the age of the person – up to 5 drops for children and up to 12 drops for adults.

On a handkerchief or kleenex tissue put a few drops of pure tea tree oil for inhalation during the day.

Put a drop of pure tea tree oil on your pillow, just under where you rest your nose, at night.

If the person is in too weakened a state to take a bath, give them a sponge bath. Use a soft face cloth, soaked in tepid water that you have added a few drops of pure tea tree oil to.

Drink plenty of water and a commercially prepared tea tree oil herbal tea – either hot or as a refreshing ice cold tea. The drink can soothe your throat and may help stimulate your immune system.

Fleas – see Insect Bites

Flu – see Bronchial Congestion, Colds, Congestion, Coughs, Fever, Aches and Pains, Sinusitis, Sore Throat

Flu, also known as influenza, is an acute contagious viral disease, characterized by inflammation of the respiratory tract, fever and muscular pain. Respiratory symptoms could include a sore throat, catarrh or a dry cough.

Preventing or reducing the severity of an attack of flu, is effectively done with tea tree oil.

Recommendations

Inhalation using a vaporizer is very beneficial. Use vaporizers throughout the home, during the illness and particularly at the beginning. Put 5 drops of pure tea tree oil into the water in your vaporizer and make sure to use the vaporizer in the bedroom at night. Boost the benefits by adding 2-3 drops of pure tea tree oil to 1 tsp (1/6 oz, 5 ml) of eucalyptus oil and put this mixture in the vaporizer or add the tea tree oil and eucalyptus oil mixture to 2 cups (16 oz, 473 ml) of boiling water to freshen and add healing benefits to the air. Another inhalation formula we have found very helpful is 3 drops of tea tree oil, 3 drops of essential oil of lavender and 3 drops of essential oil of eucalyptus.

To relieve congestion, add 5-6 drops of pure tea tree oil, to a pot or bowl of boiling water. If using a facial steamer add 2-3 drops with water, into the reservoir. Drape a towel over your head and the container. For 5-10 minutes breathe the steam in deeply. Repeat at least twice a day.

Note Viruses are usually destroyed by very hot steam.

On a handkerchief or kleenex tissue put a few drops of pure tea tree oil for inhalation during the day.

At night put a drop of pure tea tree oil on your pillow, just below your nose.

For a sore throat, gargle at least 2-3 times daily with a solution of 4-6 drops of pure tea tree oil in a 1 cup (8 oz, 237 ml) of warm water. Before gargling make sure you mix it well. You may use your regular mouthwash by adding pure tea tree oil to it. Most mouthwashes contain alcohol. Add 2-3 drops of pure tea tree oil per 1 oz of the mouthwash. The more alcohol content it has, the easier the oil will dissolve and stay evenly dispersed in it. Shake bottle each time before gargling.

For a cough, massage the chest and upper back with this concentrated mixture: Add 5 drops of pure tea tree oil to 1 tsp

(1/6 oz, 5 ml) of a base oil such as apricot kernel, sweet almond oil, corn, grapeseed, hazelnut, peanut, soya, safflower, sunflower, etcetera. Shake or mix the contents before each application. A little will go a long way. Apply at least twice daily.

Massage upper back and chest with a blend of 2.5% pure tea tree oil (9 drops) and 1 tbsp (1/2 oz, 15 ml) Friar's Balsam (Active ingredients: Benzoin, aloe, storax, Tolu balsam. Inactive ingredients: Alcohol). Repeat twice a day. You can use the same mixture in your humidifier. It relieves bronchial congestion and has numerous other benefits.

Drink a commercially prepared tea tree oil herbal tea – either hot or as a refreshing ice cold tea. The drink can soothe your throat and may help stimulate your immune system. Drink 2 to 8 times a day.

For aches and pains, soak in a hot bath. Add 8-12 drops of pure tea tree oil to the hot water when you are filling up the bath tub. Stir the water once the tub is full. Soak for 10-20 minutes. The penetrating and pain-killing (analgesic) properties of tea tree oil increases the benefits of the hot bath. The steam helps relieve bronchial congestion.

P.S.   Try a clove of crushed raw garlic, eaten just before you go to sleep. We personally have found this helpful.

Foot odor – see Sweaty Feet

Fungal Infections of the Skin – see Athlete's Foot, Barber's
                                    Rash, Dhobi itch, Dry Cracked Skin,
                                    Jock Itch, Ringworm.

Fungal organisms are found on all healthy skin. It is when the natural balance is disturbed that an infection occurs. By taking advantage of a persons weakened immune system, infections by opportunistic fungi become present. Use the following chart to refer to the appropriate tea tree oil treatment for your condition:

Location	Fungus	Refer to
Feet	Tinea pedis	see Athlete's Foot
Face & Neck	Tinea barbae	see Barber's Rash

Location	*Fungus*	Refer to
Thigh	*Tinea cruris*	see Dhobi Itch
Groin	*Tinea cruris*	see Jock Itch
Nails	*Tinea ungium*	see Ringworm
Scalp	*Tinea capitis*	see Ringworm
Skin	*Tinea corporis*	see Ringworm

Furuncle – see Boils

Genital Herpes (Herpes Simplex type 2)

Genital herpes is an infection caused by the *Herpes Simplex type 2* virus. You can get genital herpes by being in contact, skin-to-skin, with an open sore on someone who has it. Catching it requires intimate contact, such as intercourse. It is easy to pass the virus onto other parts of the body simply by touching the herpes lesion.

Usually the first out break of genital herpes is the most severe. An indication you have it is a very uncomfortable sensation of burning sores over the genitals. The skin in the genital region becomes itchy and red and then erupts with small very painful blisters, which can last for weeks.

Once you have it, it is yours for life. It stays in a latent quiet state, punctuated by occasional outbreaks, that usually only last for a few days.

Recommendations

Wear breathable cotton clothing and do not use creams, gels or lotions that will block the flow of air to the area. Keep the area clean by washing it with a mild tea tree oil soap.

At the first sign of an outbreak take a sitz bath or wash the area frequently with a concentrated solution of tea tree oil. To 4 cups (32 oz, 946 ml) of warm water add 30 drops of pure tea tree oil. Mix thoroughly before using. This helps to prevent the infection from developing further and soothes the irritation. A sitz bath is a therapeutic bath in which only the hips and buttocks are immersed. It is normal to feel a passing warm sensation. If irritation to the area occurs, discontinue this method of using tea tree oil.

Take a shallow bath using a 15% water soluble tea tree oil solution. To make this 15% solution, mix 30 drops of pure tea tree oil with 1 tsp (1/6 oz, 5 ml) of glycerin and 1 tsp (1/6 oz, 5 ml) aloe vera juice or gel. You can use just glycerin, in which case you use 2 tsp (1/3 oz, 10 ml). For larger amounts of water soluble glycerin mixtures, the ratio is approximately 1 part of tea tree oil to 6 parts of other base liquids. Mix thoroughly. Sit in the bath and thoroughly bathe the affected area using this mixture. When using this mixture, it is normal to feel a passing warm sensation. If irritation to the area occurs, discontinue this method of using tea tree oil.

As a general disinfectant measure, add 8-12 drops of pure tea tree oil to the bath water when you are filling the bath tub. Make sure to stir the water to disperse the oil.

Apply a few drops of pure tea tree oil to blisters as soon as they appear. First, check for sensitivity. You can mix the oil with vitamin E. Apply 2-3 times a day. It is normal to feel a passing warm sensation. If irritation to the area occurs, discontinue this method of using tea tree oil. Repeat frequently for several days or until the outbreak has subsided.

Massage a blend of 10 drops of pure tea tree oil mixed with 1 tbsp (1/2 oz, 5 ml) of a cold pressed vegetable oil such as avocado, apricot kernel, jojoba, grapeseed, olive or sweet almond oil onto the affected area. Apply twice a day.

Genital Warts

Genital or venereal warts are single or clusters of rough, bumpy growths found around and in the vagina, penis, anus, groin or scrotal areas. The human papilloma virus (HPV) is the cause of this condition. Over 30 types of HPV have been discovered.

In women, these cauliflower-like soft growths can be found by the labia and vaginal opening. In men, the warts are found on their genitals. Genital warts are highly contagious and sexually transmitted.

If suspected, women should immediately have a gynecological examination and a pap smear test done with their doctor.

Two varieties of HPV are implicated in cancer of the cervix and genital.

If suspected, men should immediately seek medical attention.

Recommendations

Avoid wearing tight clothing and harsh bubble baths. Wear breathable cotton underwear. After bathing, use a hair dryer on a low setting, to keep the area dry. Keep the area clean by washing it with a mild tea tree oil soap. Do not have sexual intercourse until the genital warts are healed.

At the first sign of an outbreak take a sitz bath or wash the area frequently with a solution of tea tree oil. To 4 cups (32 oz, 946 ml) of warm water add 8-12 drops of pure tea tree oil. Mix thoroughly before using. This will help prevent the problem from developing further and soothe irritation. A sitz bath is a therapeutic bath in which only the hips and buttocks are immersed. Soak for 5-10 minutes in the sitz bath. Dry area thoroughly.

Take a shallow bath using a water soluble solution. To make this 15% solution, mix 30 drops of pure tea tree oil with 1 tsp (1/6 oz, 5 ml) of glycerin and 1 tsp (1/6 oz, 5 ml) aloe vera juice or gel. You can use just glycerin, in which case you use 2 tsp (1/3 oz, 10 ml). For larger amounts of water soluble glycerin mixtures, the ratio is approximately 1 part of tea tree oil to 6 parts of other base liquids. Mix thoroughly. Sit in the bath and thoroughly bathe the affected area using this mixture. When using this mixture it is normal to feel a passing warm sensation. If irritation to the area occurs, discontinue this method of using tea tree oil.

As a general disinfectant measure bathe daily and dry the area thoroughly. Add 8-12 drops of pure tea tree oil to the bath water when you are filling the bath tub. Make sure to stir the water to disperse the oil. If irritation to the area occurs, discontinue this method of using tea tree oil.

Genitourinary Infections – see Candida, Cystisis, Genital
Herpes, Genital Warts, Thrush.

Genitourinary infections are a general classification for infections of the genital and urinary organs. See the appropriate condition for recommended treatments. The antiseptic/bactericidal, anti-itching, antifungal, anti-viral and immune system stimulating properties of tea tree oil make it an excellent agent for dealing with genitourinary infections.

The following is an excerpt from Dr. S. Cabot's findings at the December 1990 conference proceedings on Modern Phytotherapy – the Clinical Significance of Tea Tree Oil and Other Essential Oils, at Macquarie University in Sydney, Australia. Dr. S. Cabot in his presentation *'The Use of Tea Tree Oil in Clinical Practice'* concluded, *"It (tea tree oil) will help relieve the itch from the genital wart virus, from Candida, and from non-specific bacterial or fungal infection. It will relieve the symptoms as well as overcoming the infections..."*

In 1991 the British medical journal, *Lancet*,[13] reported the findings of Dr. Blackwell of the Department of Genitourinary Medicine in Wales. He reported on a patient who used 200 milligrams of tea tree oil in a vegetable base oil (vaginal pessary) instead of using metronidazole, the standard pharmaceutical drug to treat her vaginal infection. Within six days the infection cleared up. Dr. Blackwell concluded, *'tea tree oil in the treatment of bacterial vaginitis may be a safe, non-toxic alternative to standard antibiotic treatment especially in pregnancy.'*

In 1991 the *International Journal of Alternative and Complementary Medicine*[14] reported on a study by A. Shemesh and W. Mayo in San Juan Capistrano, California. They examined the usefulness of tea tree oil in creams, as an oil and lozenges to treat herpes simplex and monila as well as a host of other conditions. In conclusion A. Shemesh and W. Mayo wrote: *'Tea tree oil offers a natural, less expensive, effective alternative to currently used drugs for the described conditions in this study. It is safe, easily accessible and its side-effects profile superior to most products currently prescribed for these medical problems.'*

German Measles – see Measles

Gingivitis – see Mouth and Gum Infections

Gingivitis is a build up of bacterial plaque that causes the gums to swell, redden and bleed easily. Tea tree oil's bactericidal action, analgesic properties and ability to soften and reduce plaque, are very beneficial for gingivitis sufferers.

A worsening condition is evidenced when the gums keep shrinking away from the teeth, pus pockets start forming between your teeth and gums, teeth are loose and fall or break off near the gums. If treatment results do not appear within a reasonable period of time, then it is time to see the dentist.

Recommendations

Gargle twice a day with this blend. Mix 5-10 drops of pure tea tree oil with a glass of warm water. Gargle until you have thoroughly rinsed the mouth.

Floss twice daily. Use a commercially prepared tea tree oil dental floss or put a drop of pure tea tree oil on the floss.

Use or create your own tea tree toothpaste. Before brushing, put a drop of pure tea tree oil on your favorite toothpaste. To enhance the benefits of tea tree oil toothpaste, a good electric toothbrush is definitely worth investing in.

Gout

Gout is a form of arthritis characterized by painful swelling of the joints, especially in the big toe. It can also affect the joints of the toes, knees, fingers and other joints. It is a degenerative joint disease.

Contributing factors that cause flare ups of gout are emotional conflict, stress, lack of exercise, improper nutrition and poor diet.

The principle benefit tea tree oil can offer gout sufferers is pain relief. In cases where bacteria may be the suspected cause of the condition, the additional benefits of tea tree oils antibacterial and anti-inflammatory properties are very good.

Recommendations

Make a massage oil using 1/4 cup (2 oz, 2 tbsp, 60 ml) of a light vegetable carrier oil such as jojoba, grapeseed or sweet almond oil and 30-36 drops of pure tea tree oil. Shake or mix the contents before each application. A little will go a long way.

In the beginning apply to the affected area 2 to 4 times daily then reduce to twice daily.

To reduce inflammation apply a cold compress using a face cloth or flannel cloth upon which you have added a few drops of tea tree oil. Also beneficial is a cold compress using clay and a few drops of tea tree oil mixed into it.

Bathing. For pain relief add 8 to 12 drops of tea tree oil to the bath water when filling the bath tub. If a thin film of oil appears, stir the water for greater dispersion. Relax and enjoy.

Groin Fungal Infection – see Jock Itch

Halitosis – see Bad Breath, Mouth and Gum Infections

Head Cold

A head cold is a common cold with congestion of the nasal passages.

Recommendations

Use vaporizers in which you put 5 drops of pure tea tree oil for the duration of the illness. Place them in and around the room, especially at night. Remember to refresh the water reservoir with tea tree oil. This helps prevent the spread of the infection and adds healing vapors to the air.

Do steam inhalation to soothe the nasal congestion, especially before going to sleep. Add 8-10 drops of pure tea tree oil to a bowl or pot filled with 4 cups (32 oz, 946 ml) of boiling water. Place the pot on a flat surface. Cover your head and the pot with a towel. Keep eyes closed. Inhale for 5-10 minutes. A facial steamer is an excellent way to do steam inhalation. Add 1-3 drops of pure tea tree oil to the water in the facial steamer's reservoir. Repeat as needed.

A steam vaporizer is excellent for night time use. Add 8-10 drops of pure tea tree oil to the water.

Massage a few drops of pure tea tree oil onto the forehead and nose, particularly the upper part of the nose beside the sinus cavities. Be careful not to get any of the oil in the eyes. If you do then flush them with cold water.

Head Lice (Pediculus humans capitis)

Lice are small wingless blood-sucking insects which cause itchy scalp. Head lice is a common and recurrent problem among day care or school children. They are easily transmitted from one child to the next. Lice lay tiny grayish-white eggs (nits) which fasten themselves to the hair, usually close to the scalp. The lice and eggs are very hard to see. They can be difficult to remove. If the eggs are not removed, a reinfestation will occur.

Most commercially prepared delousing treatments contain dangerous and harsh chemicals. Read the labels. Using tea tree oil requires a little more effort, but its non-toxic and therapeutic properties will benefit the user in many ways. The hair quality will not be damaged by the oil and actually it will improve. Tea tree oil does not destroy the eggs, but it kills lice! This means tea tree oil must be used until all the eggs are removed before they have hatched.

Recommendations

One simple solution for head lice is to cut the hair short, shampoo hair daily and use a blow dryer. The heat from the blow dryer is usually strong enough to destroy mites and eggs. Unfortunately the simple act of scratching lice infested scalp and hair catches eggs under fingernails and deposits them elsewhere, contaminating everything. Try the following measures.

At the beginning of an outbreak start using a 2-4% tea tree oil shampoo, boosted with 12-20 drops of pure tea oil per oz (2 tbsp, 30 ml) of shampoo. To make your own head lice tea tree oil shampoo, add 1/2 oz (1 tbsp, 15 ml) of pure tea tree oil per oz (2 tbsp, 30 ml) of shampoo. Thoroughly lather the hair and your entire body. Leave it on for 10-15 minutes, then rinse. Shampoo and lather body daily as a preventative, until the condition is resolved. Lice thrive on body hair. Lice are called crabs when they infest the pubic area.

Apply pure tea tree oil or this water soluble glycerin solution to the scalp and hair. To make the water soluble solution, first put 1 oz (2 tbsp, 30 ml) of glycerin in a container, then add 1/2 oz (1 tbsp, 15 ml) of pure tea tree oil. Seal and shake the container then add 1/2 oz (1 tbsp, 15 ml) of water. Tightly seal the container. Shake the mixture vigorously. Massage it into the scalp and hair. Wrap the scalp in a hot towel or shower cap for 10 to 15 minutes. Remove the head wrap. Shampoo then rinse. Repeat this daily until the infestation is gone.

A good scalp rub is a grain alcohol based mixture of 100 drops (1 tsp, 5 ml) of pure tea tree oil added to 1 oz (2 tbsp, 30 ml) of vodka. Shake vigorously until the oil is thoroughly dispersed in the solution, then add 3 oz (6 tbsp, 90 ml) of water to the mixture. Shake vigorously before each use to make sure the oil is well dispersed in the solution. Leave it on for at least an hour, if possible overnight, then wash it out. Use a fine tooth comb to remove the eggs. Until the condition clears up, repeat the scalp rub every 3 days. If the skin becomes irritated replace the grain alcohol based rub with one using a light vegetable base oil (jojoba, sweet almond oil, grapeseed, corn) mixture of 20 drops of pure tea tree oil to 1 tsp (1/6 oz, 5 ml) of light vegetable oil. Caution should be exercised with alcohol based mixtures. They should not be used on irritated skin. Between scalp rubs, wash hair daily with a 2-4% tea tree oil shampoo, leaving it on for 10-15 minutes before washing it out. Add a few drops of tea tree oil to a conditioner or the final water before rinsing.

To guard against continued infection, soak brushes, combs and other contaminated materials in the scalp rub grain alcohol mixture or add a few drops of tea tree oil to the rinse water. Do not borrow or lend these items to any one. In public places and schools, where lice are a problem, make sure to wash your hands frequently.

Even though there is a question as to whether or not lice and their eggs will survive and nest in fabrics and cause reinfection, it is an inexpensive precaution to add 20-30 drops of tea tree oil when doing the laundry.

Hemorrhoids – see Piles, Varicose Veins

A hemorrhoid is a varicose vein in the anus or rectum that can cause a lot of pain – burning, itching and sometimes throbbing pain. Occasionally bleeding occurs, which is when you should seek medical help to make sure that it is a hemorrhoid, not another problem that can be related to rectal bleeding. Trust us, it really works! We have used it on and off for years – so to speak. (That's what is called 2/3rds of a pun – PU! We just couldn't resist sneaking in a bit of humor, considering the bum nature of this problem. Ouch!)

Recommendations

Gently wipe the area clean. Put a few drops of pure tea tree oil on a cotton ball or on your finger. Apply to the hemorrhoids. Repeat as needed.

Apply petroleum jelly (Vaseline). Blend 15-20 drops of pure tea tree oil with 1 tbsp (1/2 oz, 15 ml) of petroleum jelly. Mix thoroughly. Gently wipe the area clean. Dab a little of the mixture onto a cotton ball or a finger tip, then apply to the problem area. Repeat as needed.

Apply a tea tree oil and Zinc Ointment (active ingredient: 15% zinc oxide – inactive ingredients: anhydrous lanolin, cetostearyl alcohol, paraffin, white petroleum) or Ihle's Paste (active ingredients: zinc oxide – inactive ingredients: lanolin, starch, white petroleum) combination. These two zinc oxide based products are inexpensive and available at drugstores. Blend 15-20 drops of pure tea tree oil with 1 tbsp (1/2 oz, 15 ml) of Zinc Ointment or Ihle's Paste. The astringent nature of zinc oxide, combined with the healing and cleansing properties of tea tree oil are very beneficial to the pain and swelling caused by hemorrhoids. Gently wipe the area clean. Dab a little of the mixture onto a cotton ball or finger tip, then apply to the problem area. Repeat as needed.

You can mix the petroleum jelly and zinc oxide ointments (Ihle's Paste is a premixed combination of both) blended with tea tree oil together.

Take a therapeutic sitz bath, in which only the hips and buttocks are immersed. Fill the bath with 3-4 inches (7.5-10 cm) of warm water, add 20-24 drops of pure tea tree oil. Mix thoroughly before using. The sitz bath relaxes the anal sphincter muscles, taking pressure off the tender spots. The tea tree oil adds pain-killing and healing benefits to the sitz bath. It helps prevent infection and soothes the irritation. Soak for 15-20 minutes in the sitz bath. Repeat as needed.

Herpes Simplex type 1 – see Cold Sores

Herpes Simplex type 2 – see Genital Herpes

Hives – see Nettle Rash, Urticaria.

Hives are an allergic skin condition or hypersensitive reaction characterized by itching, burning and the formation of smooth patches. This type of reaction can be triggered by numerous factors such as foods, and irritants such as dust, stress, dust mites, etcetera. Determine and avoid the source.

For cases of chronic hives consult with your health care provider to determine the source and an appropriate course of action.

Recommendations

Massage a few drops of pure tea tree oil into the affected area.

For larger areas make a water-based lotion. Add 23-24 drops of pure tea tree oil to 1/2 cup (4 oz, 118 ml) of distilled or cold boiled water. Shake vigorously before each application. Apply twice daily to the affected area.

Apply this soothing and healing lotion. Mix 2 tbsp (1 oz, 30 ml) of distilled witch hazel (Hamamelis water) and 6-8 drops of tea tree oil. Shake lotion vigorously before applying to skin. Apply to the affected area as needed.

Wash with a tea tree oil soap, or add 1-3 drops to a soapy face cloth using a non-allergenic or 100% glycerin soap your health care provider or pharmacist recommends.

To bath water add 8-12 drops of pure tea tree oil. Mix it in thoroughly.

To bath water add a water soluble glycerin base mixture. In a container, first put 2 oz (4 tbsp, 60 ml) of vegetable glycerin add

1 oz (2 tbsp, 30 ml) of pure tea tree oil and 1 oz (2 tbsp, 30 ml) of water or aloe vera. Tightly seal the container. Finally, shake the mixture vigorously then add to the bath water.

Moisturize your skin by massaging a tea tree oil moisturizer in the affected areas. If you are using a moisturizer already, add a few drops of pure tea tree oil to it to increase its effectiveness.

Hepatitis – see Immune System

Hepatitis is an inflammation of the liver. The most common forms are hepatitis A and hepatitis B. Both of these are caused by a virus and are contagious.

Horseflies – see Insect Bites

Immune System (to Strengthen)

The immune system is what protects the body from damage due to infection, disease or other traumas that can harm the body. Three groups of cells (the 'T' and 'B' cells and the phago-cytes) work together to defend the body. These cells come from white blood cells in the bone marrow. The nervous system, lymphatic drainage system and other body functions work in partnership with the immune system to help the body function optimally.

Damage to the immune system makes the body susceptible to invasion from disease bearing, pathogenic organisms.

Suppressed immune systems and viral infections are becoming more of a problem. Diseases such as Chronic Fatigue Syndrome, AIDS and other infections caused by viruses are showing symptoms not previously experienced.

In Australia, tea tree oil is being used by medical practitioners as a preventative measure before surgery to increase their patients immune system response, also to strengthen the immune system of people who have long term chronic illnesses, such as hepatitis, Chronic Fatigue Syndrome, glandular fever, etcetera.

In a 1988 feature article on AIDS, in the *International*

Journal of Aromatherapy, they presented information about some success with investigations into slowing down the development and treatment of AIDS using tea tree oil.

Tea tree oil is very beneficial, because of its wide range of therapeutic properties that help the body fight and resist infection. Here is how:

- by promoting the immune systems ability to build up resistance.
- by helping the cells and organs involved, to become stimulated and more active in the healing process.
- by fighting the microorganisms that are attacking or threatening the body's normal balance.

Recommendations

Bathe at least 2-3 times a week to build up your resistance levels. Add 8-12 drops of pure tea tree oil to the bath water when you are filling the bath tub. Make sure to stir the water if a thin film of oil appears on top. In addition, you get the secondary benefit of inhalation of the tea tree oil vapors.

Strengthen the immune system by having or doing a full body massage to yourself, at least once a week, with a 2-3 per cent tea tree oil blend. Add 18-21 drops of pure tea tree oil to 2 tbsp (1 oz, 30 ml) of a carrier base oil. Use a cold pressed light vegetable oil such as avocado, apricot kernel, jojoba, grapeseed, olive or sweet almond oil. Mix thoroughly. Apply to the whole body at least once a week. Another option is to use a concentrated 4-6% tea tree oil massage blend. Add 18-21 drops of pure tea tree oil to 1 tbsp (1/2 oz, 15 ml) of a carrier base oil mentioned above. Massage this concentrated blend into the soles of your feet and palms of your hands, daily.

Inhalation of tea tree oil can be beneficial. Put a few drops of pure tea tree oil into an aromatherapy air vapor diffuser, such as a ceramic or metallic ring that goes over a light bulb. In dry climates use a humidifier or vaporizer at home and in the bedroom at night.

If you are in the hospital use tea tree oil as a disinfectant. Put 10-15 drops of tea tree oil in a clean spray bottle filled with distilled water. Shake vigorously before using. Spray a mist on the bed sheets, pillow, sink, bath room and in the area.

On a handkerchief or kleenex tissue put a few drops of pure tea tree oil for inhalation during the day.

Healing from the inside out, means using the bodies natural wisdom to heal itself. Drink a tea tree oil herbal tea – either hot or as a refreshing ice cold tea. Use a commercially prepared tea tree herbal tea. The essential oil from the tea tree is an immune system stimulant and may help.

Impetigo

Impetigo is an highly contagious skin disease with eruptions of pustules, pus filled blisters or pimples. The infection mainly affects children. It is usually caused by the *streptococcus* or *staphylococcus bacteria*. The appearance of spots or inflamed patches is normally seen on the scalp, neck and face. Sometimes blisters that crust over appear on the knees and hands.

To prevent the infection from spreading to other parts of the body, or other people, strict personal hygiene is critical.

Recommendations

Apply pure tea tree oil to the affected area using a cotton swab or the tip of a finger. Apply twice a day.

Apply this protective, soothing, healing and drying lotion. To 2 tbsp (1 oz, 30 ml) of calamine lotion add 5-10 drops of tea tree oil (for children use 5 drops). Shake lotion vigorously before applying to skin. Apply 3-4 times daily. Tea tree oil boosts the effectiveness of this lotion by increasing it's soothing and antibacterial benefits.

As a disinfectant measure, add 8 to 12 drops (no more than 5 for children's baths) of pure tea tree oil to the bath water while the bath tub is filling up. Stir water to disperse the oil. Soak and relax in the bath tub for 5-10 minutes.

Influenza – see Flu

Ingrown Nails – see Ingrown Toenail

Ingrown Toenail

An ingrown toenail occurs when the nail grows into the soft tissue, around it, rather than growing outward. The nails cutting action produces redness, swelling and sometimes infection. It is a very painful condition. Usually it occurs with the big toe.

Recommendations

The best way to deal with ingrown nails is to cut the nail straight across. This is also the best preventative measure you can take. Wear good fitting shoes.

Soak foot in a warm water bath. Add 8-12 drops of pure tea tree oil to the water. Mix it into the water. Soak foot long enough to soften the nail and reduce the pain in your foot. Use a good quality nail clipper or long handled scissors to trim the nail. Dab a drop of pure tea tree oil on the spot and on an adhesive gauze bandage or band-aid to cover and protect the area.

If an infection has occurred, rub pure tea tree oil on the affected area, two or more times a day, as needed. Tea tree oil is a very powerful germicide. It is even more effective in the presence of pus. Follow the above instructions for '*Soak Foot in Warm Water Bath.*'

See a podiatrist (foot specialist) or health care practitioner if the problem is not resolved or you have a health condition such as diabetes that warrants extreme caution with any foot infections. Bring this book and a bottle of tea tree oil with you!

Insect Bites – General guidelines

For additional information see Bee Stings, Mosquitoes, Fleas, Horseflies, Jellyfish, Sandflies, Spider Stings and Wasp Stings.

Insect bites and stings get fast relief using tea tree oil. It relieves pain, soothes itching, prevents infection from becoming a problem, particularly in children who tend to scratch the affected area.

If you have an allergic reaction to bee bites or stings seek medical help immediately. Have your health care provider prescribe an emergency treatment kit.

Recommendations

Preventative measures:

As an insect repellent, tea tree oil is very effective. The tea tree cutters and harvesters quickly discovered this, since the trees are generally found in swampy insect infested areas.

For preventative use, apply pure tea tree oil to exposed skin and clothing such as scarves, socks, collars and cuffs of shirts. For larger areas of skin apply the following oil and tea tree mixture: Add 15-18 drops of pure tea tree oil to 1/8 cup (1 oz, 2 tbsp, 60 ml) of a cold pressed light vegetable carrier oil such as sweet almond or corn oil. For up to 10% of the base carrier oil's volume you can use avocado pear, borage, carrot, evening primrose, jojoba, sesame or wheat germ oils. Shake or mix the contents well before each application. A little will go a long way. Apply as needed.

Use pure tea tree oil to keep insects out of tents, homes and other accommodations. Apply pure tea tree oil to hanging ribbons or use it in a vaporizer.

What to do once bitten or stung:

Apply a drop of pure tea tree oil to the affected area, every 3-4 hours or as required.

Add 8 to 12 drops of pure tea tree oil to bath water, while the bath tub is filling up with water. Stir water to disperse the oil. Soak and relax in the bath tub for at least 10 minutes.

Apply this soothing and healing lotion to the affected area. To 2 tbsp (1 oz, 30 ml) of distilled witch hazel (Hamamelis water) add 15-20 drops of tea tree oil (for children use 5 drops). Shake lotion vigorously before applying to skin. Apply 3-4 times daily. Tea tree oil boosts the effectiveness of this lotion and adds protection against infection.

Apply this protective, soothing, healing and drying lotion to the affected area. To 2 tbsp (1 oz, 30 ml) of calamine lotion add 15-20 drops of tea tree oil (for children use 5 drops). Shake lotion vigorously before applying to skin. Apply 3-4 times daily. Tea tree oil boosts the effectiveness of this lotion and adds protection against infection.

Itching

For those due to sexually transmitted infections or of the genital regions see Balantitis, Candida albicans, Genital Warts, Jock itch, Leucorrhoea, Pruritis, Genitourinary infection, Vaginitis

For those of or on the skin see Athlete's foot, Barber's rash, Candida albicans, Chiggers, Dermatitis, Head lice, Hives, Insect bites, Leeches and Ticks, Lice, Mosquitoe bites, Poison Ivy and Poison Oak, Prickly Heat, Psoriasis, Ringworm, Sandflies

Jellyfish – see Insect Bites

Some jellyfish stings greatly benefit from using pure tea tree oil. First remove the jellyfish tentacles using a credit card to scrap it off. Do not use tweezers or your fingers to pull out the tentacles, because you will be squeezing more venom into your skin. The embedded tentacles keep delivering a painful venom. Only the South Pacific box jellyfish venom is potentially fatal. Immediately seek medical help, if you experience vomiting, nausea, intense swelling or difficulty breathing.

Jock Itch – see Fungal Infections

Jock itch is a fungal infection of the male groin area. It is a contagious infection caused by the fungus, *Tinea cruris,* and is commonly characterized by red, flaky or soggy skin and itching. The area may become covered in a white scaly skin. The fungus can also affect fingers and nails. Numerous studies have indicated the benefits of tea tree oil when used for jock itch.

Recommendations

Bathe groin with an antifungal soap or tea tree oil soap. Dry groin thoroughly then apply pure tea tree oil or 10-20 drops of pure tea tree oil mixed with 1 tbsp (1/2 oz, 5 ml) of sweet almond oil as a base oil. You can use carrot oil for up to 10% of the carrier base oil. Once in the morning and before bedtime massage a few drops of pure tea tree oil into the area affected by the fungus. If application of pure tea tree oil to the groin area causes pain, discontinue using it and try another brand. If the condition is chronic more applications during the day may be required. Continue until condition clears up.

Apply this mixture. Mix 1 tbsp (1/2 oz, 15 ml) of isopropyl alcohol and 2 tbsp (1 oz, 30 ml) of pure tea tree oil. Shake vigorously. Let bottle rest on a flat surface for a couple of minutes. If tea tree oil floats to the surface add more alcohol and shake again, until the oil is evenly dispersed in the mixture. Store it in a glass bottle and cool place. This quantity will last for quite a while and can be used as a disinfectant.

Soak in a bath of 5-10 drops of pure tea tree oil and warm water, for 5-10 minutes each day. Dry groin thoroughly using an absorbent towel or a hair dryer.

As a preventative measure add 8 to 12 drops of pure tea tree oil to the bath water when you are filling the bath tub.

Leeches

A leech is a bloodsucking worm living in water. Today this parasite is used in modern medicine to increase the blood flow to areas where limbs have been reattached. Everything old is new again. Will wonders never cease!

The early harvesters of the tea tree discovered the plants ability to remove or repel leeches. Leeches are extremely difficult to remove, once they attach themselves to the skin.

Recommendation

Apply pure tea tree oil onto the leech and skin surrounding it. After 20-30 minutes or longer, by hand you can carefully remove those that have not already fallen off.

For at least a week keep applying pure tea tree oil to the leech bites 3-4 times daily. This prevents infection and soothes irritation.

Tip   A preventative measure you can use in leech infested water, is to put pure tea tree oil on your socks, clothing and skin areas that are exposed to the leeches. This acts as a repellent and is what the early harvesters did to ward off leeches in swampy locations where the Melaleuca alternifolia tree grew.

Lice – see Head Lice

Leg Ulcers

A leg ulcer is an open sore on the leg, discharging pus.

Recommendations

Prevention is the best route to go. On a daily basis, massage areas prone to leg sores before they becomes leg ulcers. Use a 5% dilution of tea tree cream or oil. To make your own 5% dilution blend 15 drops of pure tea tree oil with 1 tbsp (1/2 oz, 15 ml) of a good base cream or one of these cold pressed light vegetable oils – sweet almond, apricot kernel, corn, grapeseed, hazelnut, peanut, safflower, soya, sunflower. For up to 10% of the base carrier oil's volume, you can use borage, carrot, evening primrose, jojoba, extra virgin olive, sesame or wheat germ oils. Shake or mix the contents well before each application. A little will go a long way. Apply daily on the lower legs.

Massage a few drops of pure tea tree oil into the leg ulcer 2-4 times daily. If the area becomes irritated use one of the dilutions in this section or try another brand of pure tea tree oil.

Moisturize your skin by massaging a tea tree oil moisturizer in the affected areas, every day. To make your own blend add 15 drops of pure tea tree oil to 1 tbsp (1/2 oz, 15 ml) of a non-allergenic moisturizer to increase its effectiveness. Apply daily.

Gently bathe the ulcer sore using this mixture: Add 3-5 drops of pure tea tree oil to a bowl of boiled or distilled water. Then gently massage a 10% tea tree oil moisturizer on the lower legs. For a 10% blend add 30 drops of pure tea tree oil to 1 tbsp (1/2 oz, 15 ml) of a good moisturizing cream.

Leucorrhoea – see Itching, Pruritis

Leucorrhoea is an inflammation of the vagina that is caused by an excessive amount of bacteria or fungi. There are many ways this can happen. Often there is a thick yellow or white discharge accompanied by severe itching to the vagina.

Recommendations

Avoid wearing tight clothing and harsh bubble baths. Wear breathable cotton clothing. Avoid alcohol, coffee, tea and spices. Keep the area clean by washing it with a mild tea tree oil soap.

At the first sign of an outbreak take a sitz bath or wash the area frequently with this solution of tea tree oil. To 4 cups (32 oz, 946 ml) of warm water add 8-12 drops of pure tea tree oil. Mix thoroughly before using. This will help prevent the infection from developing further and soothe the irritation. A sitz bath is a therapeutic bath in which only the hips and buttocks are immersed. Soak for 5-10 minutes in the sitz bath.

Take a shallow bath using this water soluble solution: In a container first put 2 oz (4 tbsp, 60 ml) of vegetable glycerin then add 1 oz (2 tbsp, 30 ml) of pure tea tree oil and 1 oz (2 tbsp, 30 ml) of water or aloe vera juice or gel. Tightly seal the container and shake the mixture vigorously. Add 1 oz (4 tbsp, 60 ml) of the solution to the bath water. Mix thoroughly. If the problem is acute, add 3-5 more drops of pure tea tree oil to the water. Sit in the bath tub and thoroughly bathe the affected area. It is normal to feel a passing warm sensation. If irritation to the area occurs, discontinue this method of using tea tree oil.

Bathe daily as a general disinfectant measure. Add 8-12 drops of pure tea tree oil to the bath water when you are filling the bath tub. Make sure to stir the water before entering the bath tub.

Use a 1% tea tree oil ointment. Blend 3 drops of pure tea tree oil with 1 tbsp (1/2 oz, 15 ml) of an appropriate non-allergenic cream base. Apply as required to the affected area.

Measles

Measles (Red measles – *rubeola virus*) is an acute, infectious, communicable viral disease, usually of children. It is characterized by small, red spots on the skin, high fever, sore throat, barking cough, tiny white spots on the throat and mouth, and sensitivity to light. The rash usually starts on the face and neck area extending itself down to the trunk and limbs.

A similar, but milder type is called German measles. It is

caused by the *rubella virus*.

Teenagers, adults and particularly pregnant women should always see a doctor, as measles can lead to complications. The following suggestions, can lessen the impact and shorten the duration of an attack.

Recommendations

Reduce high fever by sponging down the body regularly, applying cold compresses, or submerging the body in a luke-warm bath to which you add 8-10 (for children 2-4 drops, and they must be closely supervised to make sure they do not get it in their eyes or mouth) drops of pure tea tree oil. Add tea tree oil when you are running the water to fill the bath tub. This helps disperse it in the water.

Use vaporizers in which you add 5 drops of pure tea tree oil to the water for the duration of the illness. Place them in and around the room. Remember to refresh the water reservoir with tea tree oil. This helps prevent the spread of the infection and adds viral fighting vapors to the air.

Do steam inhalation to soothe coughing. Add 5-7 drops of pure tea tree oil to a bowl or pot filled with 4 cups (32 oz, 946 ml) of boiling water. Place pot on a safe flat surface and cover your head and the pot with a towel. Keep eyes closed. Inhale for 5-10 minutes. A facial steamer is an excellent way to do steam inhalation. Add 1-3 drops of pure tea tree oil with water into the reservoir. Repeat as needed.

For a sore throat gargle for a few minutes with a mixture of 5-10 drops of pure tea tree oil added to 1 cup (8 oz, 237 ml) of warm water. Make sure you mix it well before gargling.

Apply this soothing and healing lotion. Mix 4 tbsp (2 oz, 60 ml) of distilled witch hazel (Hamamelis water) and 5-8 drops of tea tree oil. Shake lotion vigorously before applying to skin. Apply repeatedly to the affected area using a gauze cloth or cotton ball.

Note   This is not recommended for young babies. Consult your doctor first.

Miliaria – see Prickly Heat

Moniliasis or Monila albicans – see Candida, Thrush,
Vaginal Infections

Mosquitoes Bites – see Insect Bites

Mosquitoes bites get fast relief with tea tree oil. It relieves the
pain, soothes itching and prevents infection from becoming a
problem, particularly in children who tend to scratch the affected
areas.

Recommendations

Apply a drop of pure tea tree oil to the affected area, every
four hours or as required.

Add 8 to 12 drops of pure tea tree oil to the bath water while
the bath tub is filling up. Stir water to disperse the oil. Soak and
relax in the bath tub for at least 10 minutes.

Apply this soothing and healing lotion. To 2 tbsp (1 oz, 30
ml) of distilled witch hazel (Hamamelis water) add 15-20 drops
of tea tree oil. Shake lotion vigorously before applying to skin.
Apply to the affected area 3-4 times daily. Tea tree oil boosts the
effectiveness of this lotion and adds protection against infection.

Apply this protective, soothing, healing and drying lotion. To
2 tbsp (1 oz, 30 ml) of calamine lotion add 15-20 drops of tea
tree oil (for children use 5 drops). Shake lotion vigorously before
applying to skin. Apply to the affected area 3-4 times daily. Tea
tree oil boosts the effectiveness of this lotion and adds protection
against infection.

Tea tree oil is an effective mosquito repellent. The tea tree
cutters/harvesters quickly discovered this, since the trees were
found in swampy insect infested areas. For preventative use
apply pure tea tree oil to exposed skin and clothing such as
scarves, socks, collars and cuffs of shirts and pants. For larger
areas of skin apply this oil and tea tree mixture. To 1/8 cup (1
oz, 2 tbsp, 60 ml) of sweet almond oil add 15-18 drops of pure
tea tree oil. Shake or mix the contents before each application. A
little will go a long way. Apply as needed.

Use pure tea tree oil to keep mosquitoes out of tents, homes
and other accommodations. Apply pure tea tree oil to hanging
ribbons or use it in a vaporizer.

Mouth and Gum Infections – see Gingivitis, Bad Breath,
                                                Mouth Ulcers, Thrush

Mouth and gum infections are caused by improper dental hygiene, poor nutrition and a host of other possibilities. This results in a proliferation or imbalance of bacteria, fungi or viruses in the mouth and gums. For different problems, refer to their specific treatment recommendations. Prevention is the best method of dealing with these problems. The following guidelines are of a general nature.

Recommendations

Gargle and rinse your mouth daily with a tea tree oil mouthwash. Here are four gargling solutions you can use:

1) Buy a commercially prepared tea tree oil mouthwash.

2) Mix 2-3 drops of pure tea tree oil in a cup of warm water. Stir vigorously then gargle until you have thoroughly rinsed the mouth.

3) Gargle with a mouthwash you add pure tea tree oil to. Most mouthwashes contain alcohol. Add 2-3 drops of tea tree oil per oz (30 ml) of your regular mouthwash. The more alcohol content it has, the easier the oil will dissolve and stay evenly dispersed in it. If you see a film of oil on the surface of the mouthwash, shake it vigorously to disperse it more evenly in the solution. Shake the bottle each time before gargling.

4) Add a water soluble glycerin based solution to your mouthwash. Glycerin has a sweet taste. In a container first put 1 oz (2 tbsp, 30 ml) of vegetable glycerin add 1/2 oz (1 tbsp, 15 ml) of pure tea tree oil and 1/2 oz (1 tbsp, 15 ml) of water. Tightly seal the container. Shake the mixture vigorously. Place the jar and mixture on a flat surface and let it stand for a couple of minutes. If a thin film or drops of the oil appear on the surface, add more glycerin and shake until the oil is fully dissolved. If the container looks uniformly cloudy the tea tree oil is fully dispersed and the mixture is ready to use. Next make it into a 2 1/4 - 2 1/2% tea tree oil mouthwash by adding the above water soluble glycerin-based solution to 18-20

oz (540-600 ml) of your regular or your children's regular mouthwash. Shake vigorously. This mixture is suitable for children. Make sure they do not swallow it.

Brush frequently or at least twice a day using a tea tree oil toothpaste, or add a drop of tea tree oil to your regular toothpaste before brushing. To enhance the benefits of tea tree oil toothpaste a good electric toothbrush is definitely worth investing in.

Floss twice daily. Get a commercially prepared tea tree oil dental floss or put a drop of pure tea tree oil on the floss.

Mouth Ulcers – see Canker Sores

Mouth ulcers are caused by a minor viral infection. The tiny blisters burst and form ulcers approximately 1/50th to 1/4 of an inch in diameter (2-10 mm) on or under the tongue, or on the inside of the cheeks.

Mouth ulcers are one way your body sometimes indicates it is stressed. Help your body with nutritional support and supplementation.

Recommendations

As soon as mouth ulcers develop dab pure tree oil onto the spot twice daily for at least 3 days. Use your finger or a cotton tipped swab soaked in pure tea tree oil. (You can make a diluted mixture of tea tree oil with an equal amount of water, mix well and apply this with a cotton tipped swab.) Early treatment prevents the sores from developing any further. Repeat until the condition disappears. It may take several days.

In the initial stages before the sores break open, instead of pure tea tree oil, you can use a grain alcohol based solution. Add 6 drops of pure tea tree oil to 1 tsp (1/6 oz, 5 ml) of a grain alcohol such as vodka.

Gargle every morning and evening with a mouthwash you add tea tree oil to. Most mouthwashes contain alcohol. The more alcohol content it has, the easier the oil will dissolve and stay evenly dispersed in it. Add 3-5 drops of tea tree oil per oz of mouthwash. Shake bottle each time before gargling.

Rinse the mouth or gargle at least twice daily with a solution of 5-10 drops of pure tea tree oil in a glass of 8 oz of warm water. Mix vigorously. After brushing your teeth, gargle with the solution every morning and evening.

Brush frequently or at least twice a day using a tea tree oil toothpaste, or add a drop of tea tree oil to your regular toothpaste before brushing.

Drink a commercially prepared tea tree oil herbal tea, 2 to 8 times a day, to support your body's immune system.

Muscular – see Aches and Pains – Muscular

Naga Sores – see Ulcers: Varicose and Tropical

Nails (Infected) – see Ingrown Nails, Ingrown Toenails, Paronychia, Ringworm

A nail infection is due to a fungus. It can be caused by an immune system deficiency and is aggravated by moisture. In it's early stages it does not hurt nor is it a threat to your health. Long-term, if left untreated, it shows up as yellow, thick, raggedy-looking nails on the fingers and toes. Keep area dry and follow recommendations for Paronychia and Ringworm.

Nasal Passage (Blocked) – see Head Cold, Sinusitis

Nettle Rash – see Hives, Urticaria

Nettle rash is an eruption of spots on the skin. It maybe caused by an allergic skin condition or hypersensitive reaction, and is characterized by itching and burning.

Recommendations

Massage pure tea tree oil into the affected area.

For larger areas make a water-based lotion. Add 23-24 drops of tea tree oil to 1/2 cup (4 oz, 118 ml) of distilled water. Shake vigorously before each application. Apply twice daily to the affected area.

Apply this soothing and healing lotion. Mix 2 tbsp (1 oz, 30 ml) of distilled witch hazel (Hamamelis water) and 6-8 drops of pure tea tree oil. Shake lotion vigorously before applying to skin. Apply to the affected area.

Wash with a tea tree oil soap.

To bath water add 8-12 drops of pure tea tree oil. Add it to the running water while filling the bath tub. Mix it in thoroughly.

To bath water add a water soluble glycerin base mixture. In a container first put 2 oz (4 tbsp, 60 ml) of vegetable glycerin then add 18-20 drops of pure tea tree oil and 1 oz (2 tbsp, 30 ml) of water or aloe vera juice or gel. Tightly seal the container. Finally, shake the mixture vigorously then add to bath water.

Moisturize your skin by massaging a tea tree oil moisturizer in the affected areas. If you are using a regular moisturizer add a few drops of pure tea tree oil to it to increase its effectiveness.

Nipples (Sore)

Sore nipples caused by dry or cracked skin, respond well to tea tree oil. If breast feeding, make sure the tea tree oil residue on the skin is removed before the feeding. While tea tree oil is considered non-toxic, ingestion of pure tea tree oil is not recommended.

Recommendations

Apply a small amount of a 15% tea tree oil water soluble glycerin mixture to the area. To make this 15% solution, mix 30 drops of pure tea tree oil with 1 tsp (1/6 oz, 5 ml) of glycerin and 1 tsp (1/6 oz, 5 ml) aloe vera juice or gel. You can use just 2 tsp (1/3 oz, 10 ml) of glycerin in the base. For larger amounts of water soluble glycerin mixtures, the ratio is 1 part of tea tree oil to 6 parts of other base liquids.

Apply a tea tree and wheat germ oil mixture. Mix 12-15 drops of pure tea tree oil with 1 tsp (1/6 oz, 5 ml) of wheat germ oil or a good moisturizing cream. Massage into affected area once in the morning, at lunchtime and at night until the condition improves. A preventative measure is to apply the tea tree moisturizing mixture daily.

Ovarian Cysts

An ovarian cyst is a diseased sac like structure that is attached to an ovary, the female reproductive gland that produces the eggs. In studies, tea tree oil has proven to be a very effective and safe treatment, compared to other methods. If symptoms persist, see your doctor.

Recommendations

If possible get tea tree oil vaginal suppositories through your health food store. Use as directed. It helps reduce and melt the cyst away.

Another choice is to saturate a tampon using a few drops of undiluted pure tea tree oil or add 8-12 drops of pure tea tree oil to a glass of sterilized water (boiled). Mix it, let it cool, and then saturate the tampon with it. Another mixture is made by adding 6-8 drops of tea tree oil mixed with 1 tbsp (1/2 oz, 15 ml) of glycerin. Add this to 1 cup (237 ml) of warm water. Mix. Soak tampon in water then insert in vagina. Replace the tampon every 8 hours. You may feel a slight cooling sensation.

Paronychia – see Ingrown Nails, Ingrown Toenails, Nails Infected, Ringworm

Paronychia is a fungal infection that affects toenails and fingernails. Cuticles become painful and red with a small discharge. Skin below nails becomes discolored. In it's early stages it does not hurt nor is it a threat to your health. Long-term, if left untreated, it shows up as yellow, thick, raggedy-looking nails on the fingers and toes.

Main causes are harsh detergents or using false nails too frequently.

Tea tree oils penetrating qualities and antifungal properties, make it an excellent choice for treating this condition.

Recommendation

At least 3-4 times a day, soak the infected fingernails and toenails in pure tea tree oil. Massage the pure tea tree oil into the infected nailbeds. Continue until the infection clears.

Pediculus humans capitis – see Head Lice

Piles – see Hemorrhoids

Pimples

A pimple is often a small inflamed area of the skin. It is an unsightly skin condition that is very common during adolescence and during times of hormonal upheaval, such as before and after menstruation and menopause.

The condition may be worsened by lack of proper nutrition, poor diet, not enough exercise or physical activity, poor personal hygiene, stress and emotional factors.

Recommendations

Pay particular attention to personal hygiene. Wash affected area with an hypo-allergenic unscented mild soap or a tea tree oil soap, containing at least 2% of the oil.

Put undiluted tea tree oil on a cotton swab or your finger and apply it directly to the individual spots at night before going to sleep and in the morning. If it is a particularly bad condition apply 4 times the first day and 2 or 3 times for the next 3 days.

Make a 5% dilution of tea tree oil by mixing it with a hypo-allergenic cream, gel or lotion. For 1 tbsp (1/2 oz, 15 ml) of base use 15 drops of pure tea tree oil. For 1/4 cup (4 tbsp, 2 oz, 60 ml) use 60 drops of essential tea tree oil. Commercially available tea tree ointments are available. Apply as a cleansing and moisturizing agent. Use a clean cloth each time.

Mix 1/2 cup (8 tbsp, 4 oz, 118 ml) of distilled water with 30 drops of tea tree oil. Before each use, shake the container vigorously. Morning and night bathe the affected areas with the mixture, making sure to use a clean cloth each time.

Add 8 to 12 drops of tea tree oil to your bath water. Soak and relax in the bath tub for at least 10 minutes. One advantage of this is that you also get a facial steam.

Create your own facial sauna. To a bowl of boiling water, add 3 to 5 drops of tea tree oil. Use a towel to cover your head and the bowl. Let your face enjoy the steam for 8 to 15 minutes, then gently wipe your skin with a clean cloth. Do this 3 to 5 times a week.

Plantar Warts

Plantar warts (*Veruccae plantaris*) are small, usually less than 1/4 inch, sometimes larger. They are caused by a virus invasion through an abrasion or microscopic cut on the sole of the foot. The warts grow inward and under the skin. The pressure exerted by walking causes the area to become flattened until it becomes callused and has a tiny black dot on the surface. They can be very painful. They are difficult to get rid of and may reappear.

Recommendations

Apply pure tea tree oil to the Plantar wart, 3-4 times a day. The advantages of this is that it is not painful and does not affect the healthy tissue surrounding the wart like most other treatment methods. It is also a lot cheaper to do. Patience is needed as it can take over a month to be effective.

Coat Plantar warts daily, with a 50/50 blend of pure tea tree oil and myrrh (a fragrant gum resin) resin. Cover the coating with an adhesive bandage. After a few days, the skin will appear yellowish and soggy. Then you can dig out the black dots of the virus with a sterilized needle. Apply a drop of pure tea tree oil to the needle and spot each time. This treatment takes about 5-7 weeks depending on how bad and how deep the Plantar's warts are. Continue treatment with tea tree oil until the skin is healed.

Poison Ivy – see Poison Oak

Poison ivy is a plant having leaves of three leaflets and ivory -colored berries. When the sap from the plant comes in contact with exposed skin, it causes a severe rash, redness, swelling, blistering, and intense itching in sensitive people. Reaction may take hours or days to develop. At the first sign of symptoms of poison ivy, a burning and itching sensation, take action. This may help to prevent its from developing further.

Recommendations

Massage the affected area, 2-3 times a day, with pure tea tree oil. With young children, you may want to use the massage oil mixture below.

Massage the affected area with this 10% tea tree massage oil mixture. Mix 30 drops of pure tea tree oil in 1 tbsp (1/2 oz, 15 ml) of cold pressed sweet almond or corn oil. You can replace up to 10% of the base oil's volume with cold pressed apricot kernel or carrot oil. For larger amounts of massage oil just multiply the amounts by the same factor. Here is the formula for twice the above amount. For 1 oz (2 tbsp, 30 ml) of carrier base oil add 60 drops of pure tea tree oil. Since this condition can be irritating for some time, make enough to last a few days. We suggest you store it in the refrigerator between uses. A little bit gives a lot of coverage.

Poison Oak – see Poison Ivy.

Poison Oak is a climbing vine, related to poison ivy.

Prickly Heat (miliaria) – see Dermatitis

Prickly heat is a skin eruption caused by inflammation of the sweat glands. Some factors that can cause or worsen the problem include personal hygiene, nutritional deficiencies, clothing that does not breathe, emotional or physical stresses, detergents, underarm deodorants, cosmetics, allergic reactions, etcetera. The first thing to do is identify and remove the cause of the problem. Tea tree oil helps reduce inflammation and speeds up the healing process.

Recommendations

Massage pure tea tree oil into the affected area.

For larger areas make and use a 1% tea tree oil non-oily

cream or gel. Add 23-24 drops of pure tea tree oil to 1/2 cup (4 oz, 118 ml) of a non-oily cream or gel. Aloe vera gel is easy to use and readily available. If making large amounts of a gel for future use be sure to follow the storage instructions on the bottle. Blend or mix well. If it is a gel shake vigorously before each application. Apply twice daily to the affected area.

Apply this soothing and healing lotion. Mix 2 tbsp (1 oz, 30 ml) of distilled witch hazel (Hamamelis water) and 6-8 drops of tea tree oil. Shake lotion vigorously before applying to skin. Apply twice day, to the affected area.

When washing with a soapy face cloth, add 1-3 drops of pure tea tree oil to it. Use unscented 100% glycerin soap or a quality non-allergenic soap your health care provider or pharmacist recommends.

Add 1-2 drops of pure tea tree oil to a wet face cloth to wash your underarms.

To bath water add 8-12 drops of pure tea tree oil. Add it when filling up the bath tub. Mix it in thoroughly.

Add a water soluble glycerin based mixture to your bath water. In a container first put 2 oz (4 tbsp, 60 ml) of vegetable glycerin add 8-12 drops of pure tea tree oil and 1 oz (4 tbsp, 30 ml) of water. Tightly seal the container. Finally shake the mixture vigorously then add to bath water.

Pruritis – see Candida, Itching, Leucorrhoea, Genital Warts

Pruritis or itching is a most irritating condition, generally accompanying a mild vaginal infection, such as cervicitis or trichomonal vaginitis. Dr. S. Cabot, in his presentation, *The Use of Tea Tree Oil in Clinical Practice*, at the December 1990 conference at Macquarie University in Sydney, Australia, indicated *'It (tea tree oil) will help relieve the itch from the genital wart virus, from Candida, and from non-specific bacterial or fungal infection. It will relieve the symptoms as well as overcoming the infections.'*

Psoriasis

Psoriasis is a chronic skin disease characterized by scaly, reddish patches and itching. The inflammation sometimes shows up as silvery scales that appear on elbows, knees, scalp and torso. It is not contagious. The cause is usually unknown.

Possible triggers are stress, deep-seated emotional problems, damage to skin from an accident, chafing or dryness, food allergies, vitamin deficiency, environmental influences, reaction to certain drugs and infections. In some cases it has been linked to family history.

It is important to guard against infection and lessen the affect of itching, which tea tree oil is very helpful with. You can control and lessen the impact of psoriasis on your life.

Recommendations

Massage with this healing combinations of oils. The base oils are particularly effective for psoriasis. Add 15-18 drops of pure tea tree oil to 1/8 cup (1 oz, 2 tbsp, 30 ml) of a cold pressed light vegetable carrier oil such as sweet almond or corn oil. For up to 10% of the base carrier oil's volume you can use avocado pear, borage, carrot, evening primrose, jojoba, sesame or wheat germ oils. Shake or mix the contents well before each application. A little will go a long way. Apply as needed.

Moisturize the skin. Add 5-10 drops of pure tea tree oil to 1 tbsp (1/2 oz, 15 ml) of petroleum jelly or a commercially prepared moisturizer that contains lactic acid, such as LactCare. Studies indicate these are effective moisturizers for psoriasis. Tea tree oil boosts their effectiveness.

Wash with this solution: Add 15-20 drops of pure tea tree oil with 1/3 of a cup of baking soda dissolved in 1 gallon of water. Make sure to mix the solution thoroughly. Soak a face cloth or soft flannel cloth in the solution, then wring it out and apply it to the itchy area.

To a bath, add Dead Sea salts and 8-12 drops of pure tea tree oil to sooth the skin. Mix the bath water thoroughly.

In extreme cases try this combination as a massage oil. Add 20-24 drops of pure tea tree oil to this combination of 1 oz (2 tbsp, 30 ml) avocado oil, 1 oz (2 tbsp, 30 ml) borage seed or evening primrose oil and 1 tsp (1/6 oz, 5 ml) of wheat germ oil. Apply 2 or more times daily.

Note These oils are usually used as boosters to other base oils for up to 10% of the volume. There effectiveness with tough cases of psoriasis has been excellent.

Respiratory Tract Infections – see Colds, Coughs, Fever, Flu, Sinusitis, Sore Throat

Tea tree oil is anti-viral, antibacterial, stimulates the immune system, non-toxic, soothing and helps clear mucus from the respiratory tract. Can you ask for anything more in one little package!? Refer to the above conditions that best describe your respiratory tract infection.

Rheumatism – see Aches and Pains, Gout.

Rheumatism is a painful condition of the joints and muscles. The term is used to describe a wide range of conditions including various forms of arthritis, gout and muscular or joint pain. Generally it refers to rheumatoid arthritis and gout. Rheumatoid arthritis is a chronic disease with painful swelling of joints, often leading to deformity. This is caused when the inflammatory arthritis attacks the synovial membranes surrounding the lubricating fluid in the joints. This often leads to the destruction of cartilage and tissues in and around the joints and on the bone surfaces. The damaged tissue is replaced with scar tissue in the body. The entire body is affected, as the space between joints becomes narrower, develops folds and fuses together. This results in crippling pain, fatigue, fever, stiffness, swelling and weight loss. Possible triggers and causes include emotional or physical stress, poor nutrition and bacterial infection.

Recommendations

Massage is very beneficial because it stimulates circulation and helps remove toxins from the body. Add to this tea tree oils therapeutic properties and you have a winning combination. Massage the affected area with this 10% tea tree massage oil mixture. Mix 30 drops of pure tea tree oil in 1 tbsp (1/2 oz, 15 ml) of cold pressed extra virgin olive oil. You can replace up to 10% of the olive oil's volume with cold pressed sesame oil. Both oils help rheumatic conditions. Mix thoroughly before each use. Apply 2-4 times a day.

For pain relief add 8-12 drops of pure tea tree oil to the water when you are filling the bath tub.

Ringworm – see Paronychia

Ringworm is a contagious skin disease caused by a fungus. It is evidenced by a scaly, red, O-shaped lesion that looks like the rings of Saturn. Common in dogs, cats and humans, it is easily transmitted. Prevention is one of the best methods for dealing with ringworm. Wear sandals in public showers, locker rooms and swimming pools. After swimming or showering in a public place, air drying your body and direct sunlight act as good preventative measures.

Common fungal organisms that come under the heading of Ringworm and can cause infection when out of balance with your immune system are *Tinea ungium* (Nails), *Tinea capitis* (Scalp) and *Tinea corporis* (Skin). Numerous studies indicate the power of tea tree oil in fighting fungal infections. Tea tree oil takes a few days or more to be effective.

You may want to seek medical help if the following occurs: Ringworm still persists or grows after 14 days. A baby shows signs of infection. Many lesions scattered across the body. Toenails get infected by ringworm.

Recommendations

Apply a 5% tea tree cream, gel or oil. For a 5% dilution blend 1 tbsp (1/2 oz, 15 ml) of either aloe vera gel, cream or a light vegetable oil (such as avocado, apricot kernel, jojoba, grapeseed, olive or sweet almond oil) and 15 drops of tea tree oil. For a larger amount blend 1/4 cup (2 oz, 60 ml) of either aloe vera gel, cream or light vegetable oil and 60 drops of pure tea tree oil. Apply 3 to 4 times daily. It is important to treat the area and the area surrounding the infection.

Tip   Hair growth and bald spots on the scalp can be caused by

Ringworm. After the infection is gone, to help restore hair growth, substitute pure rosemary essential oil for tea tree oil in the above 5% formula. Daily massage the mixture into the bald spot.

For cases of ringworm to the scalp, do the above and wash hair daily with a tea tree oil shampoo. Use a 2-3% commercially prepared tea tree oil shampoo. To make your own tea tree shampoo, add 20 drops (1/5 tsp, 1 ml) of tea tree oil for each oz (2 tbsp, 30 ml) of a neutral pH balanced shampoo. Here's an example for a larger volume: Add 80 drops (4/5 tsp, 4 ml) of tea tree oil to 1/2 cup (4 oz, 118 ml) of shampoo. Shake vigorously before each use.

Note   It is suggested that you vary the brand of regular shampoo you use for a base, since after extended use of the same shampoo it becomes less effective as a cleaning agent. When you finish one bottle, switch brands, then switch back to the original brand. This is due to the chemical build up that happens over time.

Apply pure tea tree oil directly for small areas. Pure tea tree oil is not recommended for babies or children under age 12. For children try the water soluble solution above.

As a routine disinfectant measure when bathing, add 8-12 drops of pure tea tree oil to the bath water when filling the bath tub. Stir bath water to disperse the oil.

Disinfect bedding, brushes, clothing, combs, etcetera by adding a few drops of pure tea tree oil to the wash water of your laundry.

Rubella – see Measles

Sandflies – see Insect Bites

Sandflies are a particularly irritating insect, generally found in sandy locations. Their small size allows them to easily get through most protective defenses one sets up. The itching and scratching they cause can create open wounds or sores.

Sandfly bites get fast relief with tea tree oil. It soothes itching, prevents infection from becoming a problem, particularly in children and adults who tend to scratch the affected areas. It relieves the pain from excessively scratched areas.

Recommendations

Apply a drop of pure tea tree oil to the affected area every four hours or as required.

Add 8 to 12 drops of pure tea tree oil to bath while bath tub is filling up with water. Stir water to disperse the oil. Soak and relax in the bath tub for at least 10 minutes.

Apply this soothing and healing lotion. To 2 tbsp (1 oz, 30 ml) of distilled witch hazel (Hamamelis water) add 15-20 drops of tea tree oil. Shake lotion vigorously before applying to skin. Apply 3-4 times daily. Tea tree oil boosts the effectiveness of this lotion and adds protection against infection.

Apply this protective, soothing, healing and drying lotion. To 2 tbsp (1 oz, 30 ml) of calamine lotion add 15-20 drops of tea tree oil (for children use 5 drops). Shake lotion vigorously before applying to skin. Apply 3-4 times daily. Tea tree oil boosts the effectiveness of this lotion and adds protection against infection.

Tea tree oil is an effective sandfly repellent. For preventative use apply pure tea tree oil to exposed skin, clothing such as scarves, socks, collars and cuffs of shirts and pants. For larger areas of skin, apply the following oil and tea tree mixture: To 1/8 cup (1 oz, 2 tbsp, 60 ml) of sweet almond oil as a carrier base oil add 15-18 drops of pure tea tree oil. Shake or mix the contents before each application. A little will go a long way. Apply as needed.

Use pure tea tree oil to keep sandflies out of tents, homes and other accommodations. Apply pure tea tree oil to hanging ribbons or use it in a vaporizer.

Salpingitis

Salpingitis is caused by the streptococci and staphylococci bacteria. It is an inflammation of the Fallopian tubes. Symptoms can include fever, vaginal discharge and vomiting. Once diagnosed it must be treated immediately. The usual treatment is antibiotics. When taking antibiotics eat yogurt with live bacterial culture or take a bacterial supplement to restore the intestinal balance of good bacteria.

Recommendation

Massage the abdomen 3 to 4 times a day with this 10% tea tree massage oil mixture. Mix 30 drops of pure tea tree oil in 1 tbsp (1/2 oz, 15 ml) of a light base oil such as jojoba, olive, apricot kernel, avocado, grapeseed or sweet almond oil. Mix thoroughly.

Other options include saturating a tampon using a few drops of undiluted pure tea tree oil or adding 8-12 drops of pure tea tree oil to a glass of sterilized water (boiled). Mix it. Let it cool. Then saturate the tampon with it. Soak a tampon in water then insert it in the vagina. Replace the tampon every 8 hours. You may feel a slight cooling sensation.

Scabies

Scabies is a highly contagious itching skin disease caused by the itch mite, *sarcoptes scabiei*. The female mite burrows under the skin to lay its eggs. The newly hatched mites burrow out of the skin and this causes severe itching and irritation. Possible signs include small red pimples and scratching, which may result in sores that can become infected. Areas commonly affected by this condition include the groin, penis, nipples and skin between the fingers.

It is very common in sheep farming areas. Easily transmitted from the wool of sheep to farm workers. Transmission of these mites happens even in the workers change rooms or handling money handled by someone infested with scabies. Close contact, between people, is not required to pass this from one person to the next.

Recommendations

Gently wash the skin, then treat the affected area with a 5% tea tree non-oily cream or gel. For a 5% dilution blend 1 tbsp (1/2 oz, 15 ml) of aloe vera gel or non-oily non-allergenic cream and 15 drops of tea tree oil. For a larger amount blend 1/4 cup

(2 oz, 60 ml) of aloe vera gel or non-oily non-allergenic cream and 60 drops of pure tea tree oil. Use 2 to 3 times daily.

As a routine disinfectant measure, when bathing add 8-12 drops of pure tea tree oil to the bath water when filling the bath tub. Stir bath water to disperse the oil.

Note To prevent reinfection during treatment, meticulous personal hygiene is critical. Change and wash all bed linens, towels, clothes, etcetera. When washing these items add a few drops of pure tea tree oil to the water. Make a 10% tea tree oil solution. Mix 60 drops of pure tea tree oil with 1/8 cup (1 oz, 30 ml) alcohol. Soak a sponge in the 10% solution, squeeze it until it is damp, then sponge the mattress. Use a cloth with the 10% solution to wash metal money (change), phones and other surfaces the infected person comes in contact with. Make sure to wash the cloth in water you add a few drops of pure tea tree oil to.

Shaving Rash

A rash is an eruption of spots on the skin, in this case caused by shaving which can lead to bacterial or fungal infections or be compounded by an outbreak of acne. To sooth and reduce irritation as well as prevent infection, tea tree oil blends are very helpful. Avoid commercial after-shaves or harsh soaps.

Recommendations

Apply this soothing and healing lotion. Mix 2 tbsp (1 oz, 30 ml) of distilled witch hazel (Hamamelis water) and 15-20 drops of tea tree oil. Shake lotion vigorously before applying to skin. Apply to the affected area.

Apply 10-15 drops of pure tea tree oil blended with 2 tbsp (1 oz, 30 ml) of aloe vera gel or juice to the affected area. Shake vigorously before each use.

Apply a 2% water soluble lotion, using 2 drops of pure tea tree oil in 1 tsp (1/6 oz, 5 ml) of glycerin. Shake vigorously before applying in the morning and at night.

Apply a 15% tea tree oil water soluble glycerin mixture to the skin. To make this 15% solution mix 30 drops of pure tea tree oil with 1 tsp (1/6 oz, 5 ml) of glycerin and 1 tsp (1/6 oz, 5 ml) of water or aloe vera juice or gel. You can use just glycerin, in which case you use 2 tsp (1/3 oz, 10 ml). For larger amounts of water soluble glycerin mixtures, the ratio is approximately 1 part tea tree oil to 6 parts of other base liquids.

Massage the face with this massage oil: Mix 9 drops of pure tea tree oil in 1 tbsp (1/2 oz, 15 ml) of a light base oil such as grapeseed or sweet almond oil. Mix thoroughly before applying. This is not recommended for those with problems caused by oily skin conditions.

Shingles – see Chickenpox

Shingles, also called Zona, is the nontechnical term for the *herpes zoster virus*, the same one responsible for chickenpox. It affects the sensory nerves causing blisters to appear, usually in a band around the trunk of the body. Sometimes it is accompanied by severe pain, a rash and possibly a fever.

Treatment is the same as that used for chickenpox.

Sinusitis – see Colds, Fever

Sinusitis is an inflammation of the sinuses. The mucous membranes that line the cavities above, behind and to each side of the nose become swollen. It may follow an attack of hay fever, a cold, or long exposure to damp air or cold. A severe attack may be accompanied by congested headaches and catarrh, occasionally fever. Long-term or chronic sinusitis is due to a mild infection. This causes the nose to be constantly blocked plus a feeling of tension or a dull pain in the area between the eyes. Repeat attacks usually indicate an intolerance or allergies to cow's milk or gluten, a protein found in wheat based products.

It is important to note that sinusitis can result in secondary infections, such as those of the ear and once in a while meningitis – the three membranes that envelop the brain and spinal column. If you are in doubt, immediately seek medical assistance.

Recommendations

Immediately start steam inhalation to prevent infection from developing any further and to relieve congestion. To a bowl of steaming hot water add 5 drops of pure tea tree oil and inhale for 5 to 10 minutes. If you want to capture more of the steam, drape a towel over your head and the bowl. Make sure the table and bowl are very stable and secure. Be very careful not to spill any of the hot water and burn or scald yourself. When using a facial steamer add 1-3 drops of pure tea tree oil to the water in the reservoir, and inhale for 5-10 minutes.

Note A blend of 1 tsp of eucalyptus oil and 20 drops of pure tea tree oil in 2 cups (16 oz, 473 ml) of boiling water, is very beneficial.

Make your bathroom into a steam room. Sprinkle some of the eucalyptus and tea tree oil on the wall of the shower. Run hot water. Close the bathroom door and sit in a small chair as you breath in the fumes.

Take a hot bath. Add 8-12 drops of pure tea tree oil to the running water when you are filling up the bath tub. The effect is similar to doing steam inhalation.

Inhalation using a vaporizer is very beneficial. Add 5 drops of pure tea tree oil to the water in your vaporizer. Use in the bedroom at night.

On a handkerchief or kleenex tissue put a few drops of pure tea tree oil for inhalation during the day.

Place a wet hot cloth, that you put a few drops of pure tea tree oil on, over the nose for 5-7 minutes.

At night, sprinkle a few drops of pure tea tree oil onto your pillow, just below where you rest your nose.

Sinus Passages (Blocked) – see Sinusitis

Spider Bites – see Insect Bites

Some spider bites are greatly alleviated using tea tree oil. Follow general guidelines for insect bites.

Sore Nipples – see Nipples (Sore)

Sore Throat – also see Colds, Bronchitis, Flu, Tonsillitis.

A sore throat is often the first sign of illness. Immediate treatment can prevent the further development of infection or aid in shortening the duration of the illness. It often accompanies other respiratory infections such as the common cold, bronchitis, flu and tonsillitis.

Sometimes sore throats are minor irritations caused by too much vocal activity (cheering, yelling, etcetera), winter's dry air (low humidity), allergens, bacteria, prescription drugs, pollutants, viruses or not enough sleep.

If a rasping cough accompanies the sore throat, depending on the nature of the illness, additional measures may be required. To determine the exact nature of the problem, see your health care provider.

Recommendations

Gargle with a mouthwash you add tea tree oil to. Most mouthwashes contain alcohol. Add 6-10 drops of tea tree oil for each oz of the mouthwash. The more alcohol content it has the easier the oil will dissolve and stay evenly dispersed in it. Shake the bottle each time before gargling.

Rinse the mouth at least 2-3 times daily with a solution of 7-8 drops of pure tea tree oil mixed well in a glass of 8 oz of warm water. Continue until the condition clears up.

Drink plenty of water and a commercially prepared tea tree oil herbal tea – either hot or as a refreshing ice cold tea. The drink can soothe your throat and may help stimulate your immune system. Do not ingest pure tea tree oil directly.

Apply a drop of pure tea tree oil to the back of your throat in the tonsil area. Put the tea tree oil on a cotton swab or the tip of a finger.

In extreme sore throat conditions, start steam inhalation immediately to prevent infection from developing any further and to soothe coughing. To a bowl of steaming hot water add 5 drops of pure tea tree oil and inhale for 5 to 10 minutes. If you want to capture more of the steam, drape a towel over your head and the bowl. Make sure the table and bowl are very stable and secure. Be very careful not to spill any of the hot water and burn or scald yourself.

Tip   If using a facial steamer add 1-3 drops of pure tea tree oil with water to the reservoir and steam away your sore throat.

Take a hot bath. Use 8-12 drops of pure tea tree oil. This encourages your body to sweat, which is its natural reaction to fever. The effect is similar to doing steam inhalation. If feverish, especially if the bodies temperature is high, use cool water in the bath.

Inhalation with a vaporizer is very beneficial. Put 5 drops of pure tea tree oil in your vaporizer, especially in the bedroom at night.

On a handkerchief or kleenex tissue put a few drops of pure tea tree oil for inhalation during the day.

Note   Consult your family health care provider, if condition is long lasting, worsens, or you are in doubt about what the problem is and what to do.

Spider Bites – see Insect Bites

Splinters (Infected)

Splinters are a common everyday occurrence causing puncture wounds to the skin. When there is an open wound or a piece of a splinter remains in the body, the chances of infection increase.

Recommendations

First, put a drop of pure tea tree oil on the area, then remove the splinter. Prevent infection by massaging a drop of pure tea tree oil into the area. It will lessen any pain and provide protection against infection.

If a piece of splinter remains embedded, the area may become infected, sore and with pus. Gently clean the area. First, use a drop of pure tea tree oil and then apply a adhesive bandage with a drop of tea tree oil on it or a clay poultice that you leave in place for 2 to 3 hours to draw out the splinter.

A poultice is a hot, soft, moist mass applied to a sore part of the body. To make this poultice blend 12-15 drops of pure tea tree oil with 1 tsp (1/6 oz, 5 ml) of a kaolin or clay base. Make sure to mix it well. This is very beneficial in dislodging the splinter as well as drawing pus from the infected area. Use a pair of tweezers to remove the splinter. Repeat this procedure until the splinter is successfully removed. Then cover the area with an adhesive bandage that you put 1-2 drops of pure tea tree oil on.

Sprains

Sprains are injuries caused by wrenching a ligament or muscle of a joint without dislocating the bones.

Recommendations

Apply this soothing and healing lotion. Mix 2 tbsp (1 oz, 30 ml) of distilled witch hazel (Hamamelis water) and 15-20 drops of tea tree oil. Shake lotion vigorously before applying to skin. Apply to the affected area. After applying the lotion cover it with a moist soft cloth. Keep area moist until relieved.

Massage the affected area with this 10% tea tree massage oil mixture. Mix 30 drops of pure tea tree oil in 1 tbsp (1/2 oz, 15 ml) of a light base oil such as jojoba, olive, apricot kernel, avocado, grapeseed or sweet almond oil. Mix thoroughly. Repeat 2-4 times a day.

Soak in a warm bath. Add 8-12 drops of pure tea tree oil to the warm water when you are filling up the bath tub. Stir the water once the tub is full. Soak for 10-20 minutes. The penetrating and pain-killing (analgesic) properties of tea tree oil increase the benefits of a bath.

Stiff Muscles – see Aches and Pains: Muscular

Stiff Neck – see Aches and Pains: Muscular

Styes

A stye is a small, inflamed swelling on the rim of an eyelid.

Recommendation

As soon as the condition occurs, place your face over a bowl of steaming water, to which you add 5 drops of pure tea tree oil, for 5-10 minutes. Keep your eyes closed. Steam vapors with tea tree oil do not usually irritate open eyes. If you want to capture more of the steam drape a towel over your head and the bowl. Make sure the table and bowl are very stable and secure. Be very careful not to spill any of the hot water and burn or scald yourself. If using a facial steamer add 2-3 drops of pure tea tree oil to the water in the reservoir and follow the directions above.

Note　Not recommended that you apply pure tea tree oil to the eye area directly. It stings and can cause irritation. If tea tree oil is accidentally applied or gets into the eyes, flush them with cold water immediately to alleviate stinging.

Sunburn – see Burns

Sunburn is an inflammation of the skin from excessive exposure to ultraviolet rays. The usual sources are the sun's rays or a sunlamp. The severity of a sunburn is explained as follows:

First-degree sunburn – reddens the skin

Second-degree sunburn – reddens the skin plus some water blisters.

Third-degree sunburn – See doctor immediately. This sunburn causes lower cell damage, fluid release and may cause breaks in the skin where bacteria and infections can enter.

Recommendations

Immediately apply pure tea tree oil. It can provide quick if not instant relief from heat rash or red and sore skin.

Apply this soothing and healing lotion. To 2 tbsp (1 oz, 30 ml) of distilled witch hazel (Hamamelis water) add 15-20 drops of tea tree oil. Shake lotion vigorously before applying to skin. Apply 3-4 times daily. Tea tree oil boosts the effectiveness of this lotion and adds protection against infection, especially if the area blisters.

Apply this protective, soothing, healing and drying lotion. To 2 tbsp (1 oz, 30 ml) of calamine lotion add 15-20 drops of tea tree oil (for children use 5 drops). Shake lotion vigorously before applying to skin. Apply 3-4 times daily. Tea tree oil boosts the effectiveness of this lotion and adds protection against infection, especially if the area blisters.

Surgery – see Immune System

Sweaty Feet – see Athlete's Foot, Ringworm

Sweaty feet can become a source of problems if not looked after. Fungal infections and odors caused by bacteria are two problems caused by this. Sweaty feet respond well to the disinfecting and deodorizing properties of tea tree oil. In addition, its gentle antiseptic scent is pleasing and refreshing. These measures deal with the problem as well as prevent future ones.

Recommendations

In the morning massage a few drops of pure tea tree oil into the soles of your feet.

Put a drop or two of pure tea tree oil into your shoes and on your socks. Buy shoes that let your feet breathe. Synthetic fabrics tend to lock in the moisture. Use cotton or all natural socks that allow your feet to breath and absorb the moisture.

Soak your feet nightly, for 5-10 minutes in a bowl of warm water, that you add 5-10 drops of pure tea tree oil to. Mix well.

Thrush – see Balanitis, Candida, Leucorrhoea/Pruritis, Vaginal Infections

Thrush is caused by the *Candida albicans* (formerly known as *Monila albicans*) organism. It is a yeast-like fungal infection of the throat or mouth. Candida albicans is normally present in the body. Only when it exceeds certain levels does it cause a problem.

In women the vagina is the most common site of infection. The symptoms include severe itching, redness and often a milky-white discharge.

Usually it is contracted through sexual contact with a partner. To avoid reinfection, it is very important that both male and female sexual partners are simultaneously and successfully treated before resuming sexual relations.

Some people are more prone to thrush than others. Usually this is a result of food allergies, weakened immune system, stress and quite commonly due to treatment with antibiotics. This is because antibiotics indiscriminately kill the bacterial flora in the intestine, which keep the candida organism under control.

When taking antibiotics it is wise to eat yogurt with active bacterial cultures or supplement with a full spectrum bacterial probiotic. Ask your health care provider what the best choice is for you.

Adjust your diet to help your body deal with the fungal infection more efficiently. Avoid substances which support the growth and maintenance of these infections. Stop consuming alcohol, bread products with yeast, cheese, sugar and vinegar products.

Nutritional support and supplementation are very important. Take good multi-vitamins with minerals and nutrients at least twice a day with meals.

Recommendations for thrush in the throat and mouth

Gargle with a tea tree oil mouthwash. Mix 5 drops of pure tea tree oil with 1/2 tsp (1/12 oz, 2.5 ml) of brandy and then add to a glass of 4 oz of warm water. Gargle vigorously, but do not swallow.

Brush frequently throughout the day using tea tree oil tooth-paste or add a drop of pure tea tree oil to your regular tooth-paste.

Drink a commercially prepared tea tree oil herbal tea – either hot or as a refreshing ice cold tea. The drink can soothe your throat and may help stimulate your immune system. Drink 2 to 8 cups a day.

Severe infections may require direct application of pure tea tree oil. Apply the tea tree oil to the affected area in the mouth and throat, with a cotton tipped swab soaked in tea tree oil or with a drop put on your finger.

Recommendations for thrush in the vagina

Use a tea tree oil infused vaginal suppository, under the supervision of your health care practitioner. A patient successfully used a tampon soaked in pure tea tree oil on. Soaking a tampon with pure tea tree oil requires care. It is important to keep the tampon clean before insertion. Use 6-8 drops of tea tree oil mixed with 1 tbsp (1/2 oz, 15 ml) of glycerin. Add this to 1 cup (237 ml) of warm water. Mix. Soak tampon in water then insert in the vagina and leave it for up to 8 hours. Repeat as per your health care practioner's advice.

In severe cases see your health care practitioner.

Ticks

Ticks are wingless, bloodsucking insects that infest humans and mammalian animals — cows, sheep, etcetera. Treatment is important as they are carriers of disease.

Recommendations

Apply pure tea tree oil onto the tick and skin surrounding it. After 20-30 minutes, or longer, carefully remove a tick that has not already fallen off, by hand.

For at least a week keep applying pure tea tree oil to the tick bites 3-4 times daily. This prevents infection and soothes irritation.

Tinea

Tinea is caused by a microscopic fungal mould. It shows itself in many ways. Use the following chart to refer to the appropriate tea tree oil treatment for conditions caused by tinea:

Location	Fungus	Refer to
Feet	Tinea pedis	see Athlete's Foot
Face & Neck	Tinea barbae	see Barber's Rash
Thigh	Tinea cruris	see Dhobi Itch

Location	*Fungus*	Refer to
Groin	*Tinea cruris*	see Jock Itch
Nails	*Tinea ungium*	see Ringworm
Scalp	*Tinea capitis*	see Ringworm
Skin	*Tinea corporis*	see Ringworm

Tonsillitis – see Sore Throat

Tonsillitis is an inflammation of the tonsils, a pair of oval masses of tissues at the back of the mouth. Usually caused by a virus or the Streptococcal bacteria.

In older children and adults symptoms include discomfort in swallowing due to a sore throat and congested Eustachian tubes.

Young children generally do not complain about a sore throat, but they refuse to eat.

Other symptoms include headache, high fever and feeling generally fatigued.

It is important to seek medical help, since improperly treated tonsillitis can lead to a chronically weakened immune system, rheumatic heart disease and strep throat.

Tea tree oils bacterial and anti-viral properties are particularly beneficial with an illness, such as this, which may be caused either by bacteria or a virus.

Recommendations for viral tonsillitis:

Gargle with a mouthwash 3 times a day. To make a mouthwash put 5 drops of pure tea tree oil in 1 cup (8 oz, 237 ml) of warm water. Gargle vigorously for a few minutes.

Drink a tea tree oil herbal tea – either hot or as a refreshing ice cold tea. It is preferable to use a commercially prepared tea tree herbal tea. Tea tree oil is an immune system stimulant.

Severe infections may require direct application of pure tea tree oil. With your finger or a cotton tipped swab dab the tea tree oil onto the affected area. Until a doctor determines if the infection is bacterial or viral, apply pure tea tree oil to the tonsils every hour.

Recommendations for bacterial tonsillitis:

The same course of treatment can be done for tonsillitis

caused by bacteria, but it is important to consult with your doctor as to the course of treatment you choose – especially with children.

Tip   For additional recommendations, see Sore Throat.

Note   See your doctor to have the infection cultured to determine if it is a viral or bacterial infection.

Tooth Ache – see Dental Plaque, Gingivitis, Mouth and Gum Infection

Home prevention is the best way to deal with dental problems. Yet no matter how diligent one is, problems like tooth aches occur due to such things as sensitivity (to hot, cold, sweets), build up of plaque, cavities, leaking fillings, uneven bite plane, food lodged in gums, improper nutrition, root exposure, thin enamel, etcetera.

Recommendations

To achieve quick relief, massage a drop of pure tea tree oil directly onto the sensitive tooth and surrounding gums. See your dentist to determine the nature of the problem.

Brush your teeth and inside of your mouth with a commercially prepared tea tree oil toothpaste or put a drop of pure tree tea oil on your regular brand of toothpaste. A good electric tooth brush, gently applied to the gums, tongue and cheeks as well as the teeth, will reduce your mouths bacterial count.

Gargle with a mouthwash you add tea tree oil to. Add 3-6 drops of tea tree oil per ounce of mouthwash. The more alcohol content it has the easier the oil will dissolve and stay evenly dispersed in it. Shake the bottle each time before gargling. Rinse thoroughly with the solution.

Use dental floss 2 times daily. Commercially prepared dental floss with tea tree oil is available or add a drop of pure tea tree oil onto the dental floss.

Tropical Ulcers – see Ulcers (Varicose and Tropical)

Ulcers (Varicose and Tropical)

An ulcer is an open sore on the skin or mucous membrane, that discharges pus.

Varicose ulcers are enlarged veins abnormally and irregularly swollen, that form on the lower legs, often as a result of varicose veins. The slightest break in the skin can cause a sore or ulcer to develop that takes a long time to heal. The aged, usually suffering from poor circulation, are very prone to this condition.

Tropical ulcers (Naga sores) frequently happen in hot, humid climates. A large painless sore develops, usually on the legs or feet, that becomes infected by bacteria.

In 1930, the *Medical Journal of Australia* featured an article by E. M. Humphrey about tea tree oil, titled 'A New Australian Germicide'. He wrote: *"The results obtained in a variety of conditions when it was first tried was most encouraging, a striking feature being that it dissolved pus and left the surfaces of infected wounds clean, so that its germicidal action became very effective without any apparent damage to the tissues. This was something new, as most effective germicides destroy tissue as well as bacteria."*

In addition to its germicidal properties, tea tree oils numerous other properties are very helpful in the prevention and treatment of lower limb ulcers.

Recommendations

Prevention is the best route to go. On a daily basis massage the area with a 5% tea tree cream or oil. For a 5% blend add 15 drops of pure tea tree oil to 1 tbsp (1/2 oz, 15 ml) of a good base cream or one of these cold pressed light vegetable oils – sweet almond, apricot kernel, corn, grapeseed, hazelnut, peanut, safflower, soya, sunflower. For up to 10% of the base carrier oil's volume you can use borage, carrot, evening primrose, jojoba, extra virgin olive, sesame or wheat germ oils. Shake or mix the contents well before each application. Apply daily to the lower legs.

Note For larger quantities, add ingredients, in the same ratios. Example: Blend 1/4 cup (4 tbsp, 2 oz, 60 ml) of a carrier base oil and 60 drops of pure tea tree oil.

Moisturize your skin by massaging a tea tree oil moisturizer in the affected areas, every day. To make your own blend add 2-3 drops of pure tea tree oil to 1 tbsp (1/2 oz, 15 ml) of a non-allergenic moisturizer to increase its effectiveness. Apply daily.

Gently bathe the ulcer sore using this mixture: Add 3-5 drops of pure tea tree oil, to a bowl of boiled or distilled water. Then gently massage a 10% tea tree oil moisturizer onto the lower legs. For a 10% blend add 30 drops of pure tea tree oil to 1 tbsp (1/2 oz, 15 ml) of a good base moisturizing cream.

Urethritis – see Cystitis

Urethritis a bacterial infection of the urethra which usually precedes an attack of cystitis. Since both conditions are intimately connected, it is important to understand the differences. How you treat one, is similar to how you treat the other.

Cystitis is a bladder infection caused by bacteria. It is more common in women than men.

A sign of cystitis is the need to urinate frequently, accompanied with a painful burning sensation while urinating and sometimes feeling feverish. The urine may look cloudy.

Proper hygiene is an important preventative measure. Women should wipe themselves, with a downward stroke, starting from the urethra toward the anus. Men should wash frequently, making sure to thoroughly clean the area surrounding and under the foreskin.

In the 1980's Dr. P. Belaiche[11] successfully treated chronic cystitis using tea tree oil. Of particular note was how effective he found Melaleuca alternifolia tea tree oil in treating chronic colibacilli cystitis. Very little irritation to the mucous membrane, absence of toxicity and high germicidal properties make it an excellent antiseptic.

Caution   Any internal application of pure or diluted mixtures of tea tree oil, should be supervised by your health care practitioner. See your health care practitioner immediately if there is pus or blood in the urine or the symptoms do not improve within a few days. If irritation occurs using pure tea tree oil, you can try another brand or discontinue use.

Recommendations

Flush your system by drinking distilled water. Wear loose fitting clothes and cotton underwear in addition to any one or combination of the following:

Swab the opening of the urethra each time, after urination, with a cotton ball soaked in a tea tree oil solution made with distilled or cold boiled water. Use a clean glass container with a good sealing top. To 1 cup (8 oz, 237 ml) of distilled or cold boiled water add 5 drops of tea tree oil. Shake vigorously each time before using, since the oil does not stay evenly suspended in water solutions. A clear sign of the oil not being dispersed in the solution is a thin film of tea tree oil appears on top of the water.

Drink a commercially prepared tea tree oil tea frequently throughout the day.

To bath water add 8-12 drops of pure tea tree oil. Mix it in thoroughly. Soak for 5-10 minutes. Frequent bathing with tea tree oil as a general disinfectant is a good preventative measure.

Take a shallow bath using a water soluble solution. To make a 15% water soluble solution, mix 30 drops of pure tea tree oil with 1 tsp (1/6 oz, 5 ml) of glycerin and 1 tsp (1/6 oz, 5 ml) aloe vera juice. You can use just glycerin, in which case you use 2 tsp (1/3 oz, 10 ml). For larger amounts of water soluble glycerin mixtures the ratio is 1 part of tea tree oil to 6 parts of other base liquids. Mix thoroughly. Sit in the bath and thoroughly bathe the affected area using this mixture. When using this mixture it is normal to feel a passing warm sensation. If irritation to the area occurs discontinue this method of using tea tree oil.

Apply a massage oil gently to the lower back and abdomen. Mix 3 drops of pure tea tree oil in 1 tsp (5 ml) of a light base oil such as jojoba, grapeseed or sweet almond oil. Mix thoroughly. Repeat 2 or more times daily.

Urticaria – see Hives, Nettle Rash

Vaginal Infections – see Candida albicans, Itching,
                                      Leucorrhoea, Pruritis
        – for a summary of studies see Genitourinary Infections.

Vaginitas – see Candida albicans, Itching,
                              Leucorrhoea, Pruritis
        – for a summary of studies see Genitourinary Infections.

Vaginitas is an inflammation of the canal from vulva to the uterus.

Varicose Veins – see Hemorrhoids, Piles,
                                    Ulcers (Varicose and Tropical)

Veruccae – see Warts

Verucca plantaris – see Plantar Wart

Warts

Warts (Veruccae) are small, usually less than 1/4 inch some-times larger, benign tumorous growths on the skin. They are caused by a virus invasion through an abrasion or microscopic cut on the face, fingers, hands, elbows or knees. They are diffi-cult to get rid of and may reappear. Sometimes they sponta-neously disappear.

Note Warts can be an indication that your bodies immune
        system is not working as efficiently as it can.

Recommendations

Apply pure tea tree oil to the wart 3-4 times a day. The advantages of this is that it is not painful and does not affect the healthy tissue surrounding the wart like most other treatment methods. It is also a lot cheaper to do. Patience is needed for the wart to dry out. It can take a few weeks to be effective.

Only if desperate! Coat really stubborn warts daily with a

50/50 blend of pure tea tree oil and myrrh resin – a fragrant gum resin available in health food stores. Cover the coating with an adhesive bandage. After a few days the skin will appear yellowish and soggy. You can then dig out the black dots of the virus with a sterilized needle. Apply a drop of pure tea tree oil to the needle and the wart each time. This treatment takes about 5-7 weeks depending on how big and deep the warts are. Continue coating the area until the skin is healed.

Wasp Stings

Wasp stings are caused by the release of chemicals from the stinger that penetrates the skin and releases its venom. Wasps do not leave a stinger in the body. If it does break off the wasp, the first thing one should do is flick the stinger off.

If you have an allergic reaction to be wasp stings, seek medical help immediately. Have your health care provider prescribe an emergency treatment kit.

Recommendations

Apply a drop of pure tea tree oil to the affected area every four hours or as required.

Add 8 to 12 drops of pure tea tree oil to the bath water while bath tub is filling. Stir water to disperse the oil. Soak and relax in the bath tub for at least 10 minutes.

Apply this soothing and healing lotion. To 2 tbsp (1 oz, 30 ml) of distilled witch hazel (Hamamelis water) add 15-20 drops of tea tree oil. Shake lotion vigorously then apply to the affected area. Apply 3-4 times daily. Tea tree oil boosts the effectiveness of this lotion and adds protection against infection.

Apply this protective, soothing, healing and drying lotion. To 2 tbsp (1 oz, 30 ml) of calamine lotion add 15-20 drops of tea tree oil (for children use 5 drops). Shake lotion vigorously before applying to skin. Apply 3-4 times daily.

Tea tree oil is an effective insect repellent. For preventative use apply pure tea tree oil to exposed skin and clothing such as scarves, socks, collars and cuffs of shirts and pants. For larger areas of skin apply the following oil and tea tree mixture: To 1/8 cup (1 oz, 2 tbsp, 60 ml) of a cold pressed light vegetable carrier oil such as avocado, jojoba, grapeseed, olive or sweet almond oil add 15-18 drops of pure tea tree oil. Shake or mix the contents before each application. A little will go a long way. Apply as needed.

Wounds – see Cuts

Zona – see Chickenpox

Zona is also called shingles. It is caused by the *herpes zoster virus*, the same one responsible for chickenpox. It affects the sensory nerves, causing blisters to appear, usually in a band around the trunk of the body. Sometimes it is accompanied by severe pain, a rash and possibly a fever. Treatment is the same as that used for Chickenpox.

CHAPTER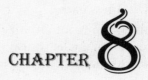

Health, Beauty Aid and Personal Hygiene Uses

For specific health problem conditions see Chapter 7 Health Uses, How to from A to Z

After Shave • Antibacterial Hand Wash • Bikini Waxing • Body Splash – Deodorizing Wash • Cleanser • Deodorant • Dental • Douches • Hair care • Make up remover • Masks • Massage • Moisturizers • Mouthwash • Sweaty Feet

After Shave – for women and men

Glycerin adds a soft emollient touch for face and leg after shaves. Tea tree oil adds cleansing and healing properties, particularly helpful for shaving razor burns or rashes. This after shave is a gentle skin conditioner, you can use daily, or once a week.

Animal glycerin, made from cattle bones, is available in drug stores. Aromatherapists and herbalists prefer vegetable glycerin, which is usually available in herbal supply shops and health food stores.

Recommendation

In a glass or clear plastic container first put 1 oz (2 tbsp, 30 ml) of vegetable glycerin, add 1/2 oz (1 tbsp, 15 ml) of pure tea tree oil and 1/2 oz (1 tbsp, 15 ml) of water. Tightly seal the container. Shake the mixture vigorously, then wait a few minutes. If a thin film or drops of the tea tree oil appear on the surface add more glycerin and shake until the oil is fully dissolved. If the container looks uniformly cloudy the mixture is okay and the tea tree is fully dispersed in it. Label the container *Tea Tree Oil After Shave*.

Use this soothing lotion. Mix 2 tbsp (1 oz, 30 ml) of distilled witch hazel (Hamamelis water) and 15-20 drops of tea tree oil. Shake lotion vigorously then apply to shaved areas.

For dry skin add 10-12 drops of pure tea tree oil to an 8 oz (1 cup, 237 ml) bottle of light mineral oil. Shake bottle vigorously. Gently massage into your skin. This combination moisturizes and helps your skin.

Antibacterial Hand Wash

To prevent the spread of disease causing bacteria tea tree oil is tops. According to research, tea tree oil kills over 99% of bacteria on contact. It does this safely and without the harshness of rigorous scrubbing that most antibacterial soaps and hand washes require, to do the job properly.

Recommendations

Add 15-20 drops of pure tea tree oil to each ounce (2 tbsp, 30 ml) of your liquid soap. Shake vigorously before each use. Commercially prepared antibacterial tea tree oil hand soaps are available.

To make your own quick drying portable lotion, that you can take with you and use in public, try this mixture. In a container first put 1 oz (2 tbsp, 30 ml) of glycerin, available at drug and health food stores, add 30 drops of pure tea tree oil and 1/2 oz (1 tbsp, 30 ml) of isopropyl rubbing alcohol or grain alcohol. Grain alcohols are less harsh to the skin. Tightly seal the container. Finally shake the mixture vigorously. If a thin film or drops of tea tree oil appear on the surface add more glycerin or isopropyl and shake until the oil is fully dissolved. If the container looks uniformly cloudy the tea tree is fully dispersed in it. Label the bottle *'External Use Only – Tea Tree Hand Wash'*.

This lotion cleans and moisturizes your hands as well as

protects you from disease causing bacteria. The alcohol helps it dry quickly. Commercially prepared ones are available.

Bikini Waxing

Before doing a bikini waxing massage 4-6 drops of pure tea tree oil on the area. Allow it to be absorbed. After the bikini waxing massage the tea tree oil lotion mixture below into the area 3-4 times the same day. This should reduce swelling and redness. An added benefit is it helps prevent ingrown hairs and infections.

Tip   If shaving your bikini line, first put a drop of tea tree oil on the razor blade.

In a container first put 2 oz (4 tbsp, 60 ml) of glycerin, available at drug and health food stores, add to it 1 oz (2 tbsp, 30 ml) of full-strength tea tree oil and 1 oz (2 tbsp, 30 ml) of water. Tightly seal the container and shake the mixture vigorously.

Test to see if the tea tree oil is evenly dispersed in the glycerin. Place the container on a flat surface and let it stand for a couple of minutes. If a thin film or drops of the oil appear on the surface add more glycerin and shake until the oil is fully dissolved. If the container looks uniformly cloudy the mixture is okay and the tea tree is fully dispersed in it. Label the bottle *Bikini Waxing Tea Tree Oil Lotion*. Store properly and it should last you a long time. This lotion can be used to rejuvenate your skin, on rough or dry hands, feet, elbows, etcetera.

Apply this soothing lotion. Mix 2 tbsp (1 oz, 30 ml) of distilled witch hazel (Hamamelis water) and 15-20 drops of tea tree oil. Shake lotion vigorously, then apply.

Body Splash – Deodorizing Wash

A tea tree oil body splash is cleansing. This one is a good deodorant since it kills the odor causing bacteria.

To 2 tsp (1/3 oz, 10 ml) of vodka add 20-30 drops of pure tea tree oil. Shake vigorously. If a film or drops of tea tree oil appear on top of the mixture add another teaspoon of vodka.

The higher the proof of the vodka, the easier the oil dissolves and is dispersed in the body splash. Next add 1/2 cup (4 oz, 118 ml) of white or cider vinegar. Finally add 2 cups (8 oz, 473 ml) of water. Shake vigorously before applying. This deodorant splash is not recommended if you have dry or sensitive skin.

Cleanser

Try this cleansing paste for all skin types. For the base oil use sweet almond or sunflower oil for oily skin, wheat germ oil for dry skin. Combine the following ingredients in a blender: 4 oz (118 ml) of base oil, 5 oz (142 grams) of ground almonds, 2 oz (60 ml) of cider vinegar, 2 oz (60 ml) distilled or spring water and 6-8 drops of pure tea tree oil. Blend about 2 minutes until you have a smooth paste. Store in a jar. Massage paste into skin and wipe off with a damp cloth. Use as needed.

Deodorant – see Body Splash Deodorizing Wash

Commercially prepared tea tree oil deodorants, that do not contain aluminum, are available. It is believed that aluminum may cause health problems with long term use. Try the body splash deodorizing formula. It may sting on recently shaved areas because of the alcohol content.

Add 1-3 drops of pure tea tree oil to a damp face cloth and wipe under the arms.

For excessive perspiration, dampen a cloth with isopropyl alcohol, add 1-3 drops of pure tea tree oil and apply as needed.

Dental Care – General

Dental care starts with prevention. Using tea tree oil products can save you time, money, reduce the cost of your dental bills as well as incidences of painful tooth, gum and mouth problems.

Reducing or eliminating dental plague build up, the bacteria ladened hard material around the teeth, is one benefit of tea tree oil. Dental plaque can affect your teeth, gums, general state of your mouth's health and health in general, if allowed to build up and remain.

In Australia dentists use a tea tree oil mouthwash to sterilize cavities before filling them. Frequent users of tea tree oil toothpaste have indicated that plaque is no longer a problem for them. One said, "My dental hygienist asked me if I had my teeth recently cleaned since the last time I had been their over a year ago." "No. Why?" I asked her. "There's hardly any plaque in your mouth."

Colgate-Palmolive in Australia tested a tea tree oil toothpaste called 'Protex'. Since it could not secure a sufficient quantity of pure tea tree oil to satisfy the potential markets it discontinued the test and decided not to produce it for commercial purposes. Several companies, like Melaleuca and Thursday's Plantation, are producing such products, making them widely available to consumers.

The following methods can help soften plaque, reduce its formation, prevent bad breath and are good for general tooth and mouth care. For specific problems, refer to Chapter 7, *Health Uses: How to A to Z.*

Recommendations

Brush frequently or at least twice a day using a tea tree oil toothpaste, or add a drop of tea tree oil to your regular toothpaste before brushing.

Create your own tea tree toothpaste. Blend in 12-15 drops of pure tea tree oil with 1 tbsp (1/2 oz, 15 ml) of your favorite toothpaste. To enhance the benefits of tea tree oil toothpaste a good electric toothbrush is definitely worth investing in.

Rinse and hold a tea tree oil mouthwash in your mouth for 1 minute. You can create your own tea tree oil mouthwash by adding 2-3 drops of pure tea tree oil per 1 oz of the mouthwash. Most mouthwashes contain alcohol which tea tree oil dissolves in. The more alcohol content a mouthwash has the easier the oil will dissolve and stay evenly dispersed in it. Shake bottle each time before gargling. This is beneficial for the gums which can be damaged by excessive bacterial plaque build up.

If you do not have or use mouthwash you can rinse the mouth with a solution of 3-5 drops of pure tea tree oil, mixed well in a glass of 8 oz of warm water. Rinse every morning and evening after brushing the teeth.

Use dental floss daily. Commercially prepared dental floss impregnated with tea tree oil is available or add a drop of pure tea tree oil onto the dental floss. This gives it an antibacterial and mildly analgesic benefit.

Clean your toothbrush once a week using a drop of pure tea tree oil while rinsing it. It helps get rid of bacteria and other infectious agents on the tooth brush.

Douches

"Daily vaginal douches with 0.4 per cent of the (tea tree) oil in one quart of water proved safe and effective in treatment of the vaginal infections under consideration." wrote Dr. E. Pena, *Journal of Obstetrics and Gynecology*, 1962. He did a clinical study of 130 women with various types of vaginal infection – Candida albicans (thrush), cervicitis and trichomonal vaginitis. He used Melaleuca alternifolia tea tree oil in a specially emulsified 40% solution of pure oil. The emulsified 40% solution of tea tree oil contained 13% isopropyl alcohol which made it possible to mix with any amount of water. A clinical cure rate of 100% was achieved. Due to the high concentration of tea tree oil he used, it is recommended that you do this with the supervision of your health care provider.

Recommendations

An easy low percentage tea tree oil douch mixture. To 1 cup (8 oz, 237 ml) of purified, cold boiled or distilled water add 8-10 drops of pure tea tree oil. Mix thoroughly before douching.

Try a sitz bath douche. To a shallow bath or bowl of warm water add 8-10 drops of pure tea tree oil. Mix thoroughly. Bathe the affected area. Soak for 15 to 20 minutes.

Try this lower body, sitz bath douche. To a shallow bath add 1/2 oz (1 tbsp, 15 ml) of this water soluble tea tree oil mixture. In a container first put 1 oz (2 tbsp, 30 ml) of glycerin, available at drug and health food stores, add to it 1/2 oz (1 tbsp, 15 ml) of full-strength tea tree oil and 1/2 oz (1 tbsp, 15 ml) of water. Tightly seal the container. Shake the mixture vigorously. If a thin film or drops of the oil appear on the surface, add more glycerin and shake until the oil is fully dissolved. The mixture is okay and the tea tree is fully dispersed in it if the container looks uniformly cloudy. Mix it into the bath water thoroughly. Sit in the bath for 5 to 10 minutes. Bathe the affected area thoroughly.

Hair Care – Daily and Dandruff Shampoos

Dandruff is a condition affecting the scalp. Overactive sebaceous gland secretions in the scalp cause scales to form, which may itch and burn.

It may be caused by poor diet, inadequate stimulation of the scalp, poor blood circulation, pityrosporum ovale yeast which lives on the scalp, Candida albicans, trichoplyton spp fungi, stress or chemical hair preparations.

Tea tree oil can clear up the problem and has an added bonus since it improves the health of your hair.

Recommendations

Blend 30 drops of pure tea tree oil with 1/4 cup (2 oz, 60 ml) of warmed coconut or jojoba oil. Massage into your scalp. If possible wrap warm towels around your head. To remove the massage oil you must first work in a 2-4% tea tree oil shampoo or blend 5 drops of pure tea tree oil with 1 tsp (1/6 oz, 5 ml) of a neutral pH balanced mild shampoo and lather into your hair. Once the shampoo is thoroughly worked in you rinse it with water. The order is very important since the shampoo helps remove most of the oil from your scalp and hair. Repeat weekly.

On a daily or regular basis use a 2-4% tea tree oil shampoo or make your own. Add 20 drops of pure tea tree oil for each oz (2 tbsp, 30 ml) of a neutral pH balanced shampoo. Here's an example for a larger volume: Add 80 drops of tea tree oil to 1/2 cup (4 oz, 118 ml) of shampoo. Shake vigorously before each use.

Note   It is suggested that you vary the brand of shampoo you use for a base, since after extended use of the same shampoo it becomes less effective as a cleaning agent. This is due to the chemical build ups that occur over time. When you finish one bottle switch brands, then switch back to the original brand.

In a rush!? A quick method you can use between washes is to vigorously massage a few drops of pure tea tree oil into your scalp and hair, then wash off with shampoo. This helps unblock the hair follicles.

Make up remover

Add 10-12 drops of pure tea tree oil to an 8 oz (1 cup, 237 ml) bottle of light mineral oil. Shake contents vigorously. Put the mixture on a cotton ball and gently remove your make up. This combination moisturizes and helps tune up your skin.

Masks

A poultice is a hot soft moist mass applied to a part of the body. It makes an excellent mask. It can be applied to the face for beauty and well-being purposes. Tea tree oil poultices can help remove dead skin and rejuvenate your skin.

To make a poultice blend 7-8 drops of tea tree oil with 2 tsp (10 ml) of corn flour and 1 tbsp (1/2 oz, 30 ml) of a kaolin or clay base depending on the skin type you are covering. Blend until it is a smooth paste. Store in a glass bottle. Particularly beneficial in drawing out the pus from pimples and infected areas. Apply to the skin leaving it there for 15 minutes. Rinse off.

If you have stubborn skin conditions make a 15 percent tea tree oil poultice. Increase the amount of tea tree oil to 15 drops for 1 tsp (1/6 oz, 5 ml) of a kaolin or clay base, .

Massage – General guidelines

Massage is one of the best things you can do for your health and general well-being. It stimulates the circulation, helps detoxify the body, increases lymphatic drainage and in addition, increases the production and release of oxytocin, a powerful natural healing chemical in the body. Combined with the beneficial properties of tea tree oil and you have a winning combination that helps keep your skin clean and healthy.

When using tea tree oil mix it with a cold pressed light vegetable oil as a base (carrier) oil. Different base oils have different properties. Cold pressed oils are mechanically extracted. They do not contain the harsh chemicals that are used in the processing of many oils, nor are they processed at high temperatures they may destroy some of the beneficial properties of these base oils.

Jojoba oil does not go rancid since it is a liquid wax. The other oils can go rancid. To prolong their shelf life add a little wheat germ oil, which has vitamin E and anti-oxidant properties, or store them in the refrigerator. Match the base oils benefits with your needs. See the accompanying chart of base oils and their properties.

How much tea tree oil you add depends on the surface area and problem you are dealing with. In the case of muscular aches and pains you may want to make a 5 percent dilution of tea tree oil – just double the amount of tea tree oil in the guidelines below. A concentration of 2 1/2 percent is sufficient for general massage purposes.

Guidelines for a 2 1/2 percent tea tree oil dilution by volume:

Amount of Carrier Oil	Drops of Tea Tree Oil
1 tsp (1/6 oz, 5 ml)	2-3 drops
1 tbsp (1/2 oz, 15 ml)	7-8 drops
1/4 cup (4 tbsp, 2 oz, 60 ml)	36 drops

20 drops of tea tree oil = 1/5 tsp (1/30 oz, 1 ml)

For massage purposes a little bit of tea tree oil diluted in a carrier oil will give a lot of coverage. Shake the contents vigorously before each application, to insure the oil is fully dispersed in it. Apply to the affected area 4 times daily at the beginning, then reduce to twice daily.

Carrier Oil Types – Benefits and Percentage to Use

The vegetable oils used should be cold pressed since this process does not use chemical agents in the manufacturing. A 10% dilution, means that the oil can be added to the base oil, up to 10% of the total volume of base oil.

A 100% dilution indicates that you can use it for part or all of the base oil volume.

Base (carrier) oils can be matched to specific health conditions which are indicated in *Chapter 7, Health Uses: How to A to Z*. Boost the effectiveness of tea tree oil by matching it with the conditions indicated for a base oil. For general massages any of the following 100% use base oils are okay.

Sweet Almond Oil

Relieves itching, dryness, soreness and inflammation
All skin types – can be used 100% as base oil

Apricot Kernel Oil

Good for prematurely aged, dry, inflamed and sensitive skin
All skin types – can be used as 100% base oil

Avocado Pear Oil

Good for dehydrated and dry skin, eczema
All skin types – use as 10% dilution with base other oil

Borage Seed Oil

Good for heart disease, multiple sclerosis, menopausal problems, PMS, psoriasis and eczema, prematurely aged skin
Stimulates and regenerates skin.
All skin types – use as 10% dilution with other base oil

Carrot Oil

Good for itching, premature aging, psoriasis and eczema. Rejuvenating and reduces scarring.
Do not use undiluted – use as 10% dilution with other base oil

Corn Oil

Soothing on all skin types
All skin types – can be used as 100% base oil

Evening Primrose Oil

Good for heart disease, multiple sclerosis, menopausal problems, PMS, psoriasis and eczema, prematurely aged skin

Helps prevent premature aging of skin
All skin types – use as 10% dilution with other base oil

Grapeseed Oil

All skin types – can be used as 100% base oil

Hazelnut Oil

Mildly astringent action
All skin types – can be used as 100% base oil

Jojoba Oil

Good for acne, hair care, inflamed skin, psoriasis and eczema. It is highly penetrative. This is the oil used by Native Americans for smooth, soft and healthy skin.
All skin types – use as 10% dilution with other base oil

Olive Oil (Extra virgin)

Good for cosmetics, hair care, rheumatic conditions. Soothing
All skin types – use as 10% dilution with other base oil

Peanut Oil (Arachis Nut)

All skin types – can be used as 100% base oil

Safflower Oil

All skin types – can be used as 100% base oil

Sesame Oil

Good for arthritis, eczema, psoriasis, rheumatism
All skin types – use as 10% dilution with other base oil

Soya Oil

All skin types – can be used as 100% base oil

Sunflower Oil

All skin types – can be used as 100% base oil

Wheat germ Oil

Good for eczema, psoriasis, prematurely aged skin
All skin types – use as 10% dilution with other base oil

Moisturizers

Moisturize your skin by massaging a tea tree oil moisturizer into the affected areas. If you are using a moisturizer already, put some in the palm of your hand and add 1-3 drops of pure tea tree oil to increase its cleansing and softening effectiveness.

For a soothing and rejuvenating moisturizer you can use daily, blend 18-20 drops of pure tea tree oil, with 1 tsp (1/6 oz, 5 ml) of vitamin E in a strength from 3,000 to 28,000 International units (available at drug and health food stores), then blend with to 2 tbsp (1 oz, 30 ml) of a non-allergenic moisturizer. Apply daily or as needed.

Moisturize your skin with this healing combinations of oils. Add 30 drops of pure tea tree oil to 1/8 cup (1 oz, 2 tbsp, 30 ml) of a cold pressed light vegetable carrier oil such as sweet almond, apricot kernel, corn oil, grapeseed, peanut, safflower, soya or sunflower. For up to 10% of the base carrier oil's volume you can use avocado pear, borage, carrot, evening primrose, jojoba, sesame or wheat germ oils. Mix the contents before each application. A little will go a long way. Apply daily or as needed.

Add 10-12 drops of pure tea tree oil to an 8 oz (1 cup, 237 ml) bottle of light mineral oil. Shake bottle vigorously. Put the mixture on a cotton ball and gently massage into your skin.

Mouthwash

You can create your own tea tree oil mouthwash by adding 2-3 drops of tea tree oil per ounce of mouthwash. Most mouthwashes contain alcohol which tea tree oil dissolves in. The more alcohol content a mouthwash has the easier the oil will dissolve and stay evenly dispersed in it. Shake the bottle each time before gargling. Rinse and hold the mouthwash in your mouth for 1 minute.

If you do not have or use mouthwash you can rinse the mouth at least twice daily with a solution of 3-5 drops of pure tea tree oil mixed well in a glass of 8 oz of warm water. Rinse every morning and evening after brushing the teeth.

Sweaty Feet

Sweaty feet can become a source of problems if not looked after. Fungal infections and odors caused by bacteria are two problems caused by this. Sweaty feet respond well to the disinfecting and deodorizing properties of tea tree oil. In addition, its gentle antiseptic scent is pleasing and refreshing. These measures deal with the problem as well as prevent future ones.

Recommendations

In the morning, massage a few drops of pure tea tree oil into the soles of your feet.

Put a drop or two of pure tea tree oil into your shoes and on your socks. Buy shoes that let your feet breathe. Synthetic fabrics tend to lock in the moisture. Use cotton or all natural socks that allow your feet to breath and absorb the moisture.

Soak your feet nightly for 5-10 minutes in a bowl of warm water, that you add 5-10 drops of pure tea tree oil to. Mix well. Soak. Aaahhhhh!

CHAPTER 9

Household Cleaning and Plant Care Uses

Tea tree oil offers many benefits for household use. It is biodegradable, environmentally friendly and safe to use. It is generally not irritating to the skin. You do not need special gloves or equipment. The fumes are beneficial. It's penetrating when used on grease, oils and other stains. It kills bacteria, molds/fungus and viruses. It's an insecticide and pesticide.

Care should be used on wood furniture as pure tea tree oil can damage some finishes. On furniture use it only in dilutions and spot test it first on an out of sight location.

Deodorizer

To deodorize a room, especially a baby's or ailing adult's room, add 3-5 drops of pure tea tree oil to an essential oil diffuser. For humidifiers or vaporizers add 10-12 drops of pure tea tree oil to the water in the reservoir. Tea tree oil also has disinfecting (anti-viral, antifungal and germicidal) and mold controlling properties, in addition to being an insect repellent. These properties are beneficial to one's well being.

Diaper Cleanser

For each gallon of washing water add 18-20 drops of pure tea tree oil. Stir water well, then soak diapers in it for 10 to 12 hours.

You can use a 15% water soluble tea tree oil solution. Mix 30 drops of pure tea tree oil with 1 tsp (1/6 oz, 5 ml) of glycerin and 1 tsp (1/6 oz, 5 ml) aloe vera juice. You can use just glycerin, in which case you use 2 tsp (1/3 oz, 10 ml). For larger amounts of water soluble glycerin mixtures, the ratio is 1 part of tea tree oil to 6 parts of other base liquids. First stir this solution into the wash water, then soak diapers in it for 10 to 12 hours. Glycerin adds softness, moisturizes and feels good on skin.

Disinfectant Uses

To disinfect a room the anti-viral, antifungal, germicidal and mold controlling properties of tea tree oil are excellent. This is very good for a baby's or ailing adults room. Add a 3-5 drops of pure tea tree oil to an essential oil diffuser. For humidifiers or vaporizers add 10-12 drops of pure tea tree oil to the water in the reservoir. An added benefit is that tea tree oil is also a room deodorizer.

Add 3-5 drops of pure tea tree oil for each ounce (2 tbsp, 30 ml) of your liquid cleaners to increase their disinfecting properties or to each bucket of water with detergent in it. If cleaners are in plastic bottles do not add more as undiluted pure tea tree oil can destroy certain types of plastics over time.

To disinfect a counter or stove top put 2-3 drops of pure tea tree oil on a damp sponge and wipe away.

You can disinfect cutting boards, kitchen utensils, etcetera by putting them in hot water containing 20-30 drops of pure tea tree oil in a regular sized sink or bucket of water. Let them soak a few minutes. Rinse, then dry off.

To disinfect laundry add 1tsp (1/6 oz, 5 ml) of a water soluble tea tree oil glycerin mixture to the wash water. Here is a water soluble tea tree oil disinfecting formula for 12 large laundry loads. To make it first put 1 oz (2 tbsp, 30 ml) of glycerin in a container, then add 1/2 oz (1 tbsp, 15 ml) of pure tea tree oil. Seal and shake, then add 1/2 oz (1 tbsp, 15 ml) of water. Tightly seal the container. Finally shake the mixture vigorously. You can add 1/2 to 1 tsp to mop water for kitchen and bathroom floors. The same formula is also good for controlling mold.

To disinfect air ducts, air conditioning units, dehumidifier collection pans, filters, humidifiers and vaporizers, spray a few drops of the water-soluble glycerin solution, using a spray mister, onto the areas you want to disinfect.

Mold

Mold is a fungus that produces a furry growth on the surface of organic matter. It can become a medium for other sources of infestation or infection.

Many children and adults are sensitive to mold, particularly those with respiratory infections. Hospitals in Australia, to keep them mold free, use air misters on timers to spray minute amounts of tea tree oil into the air, reducing the use of harsh and potentially toxic chemicals. This is a major benefit of tea tree oil. It should be considered for use in areas such as bathrooms, tubs and showers, toilets, sinks, bedrooms or any room where you come into direct or indirect contact with moldy surfaces.

Recommendations

Fill a plant spray mister with 8 oz (1 cup or 237 ml) of distilled or cold boiled water and add 6-8 drops of pure tea tree oil, depending on the nature and location of the mold. Shake bottle vigorously. Mist the affected area directly. Repeat until the mold is dead. Wipe off and remove the dead matter.

Put 10-15 drops in a room vaporizer or humidifier and let it permeate the air with tea tree oil.

If your home uses a central heating system with a built in humidifier, stir 10 to 15 drops of pure tea tree oil, for every 8 oz (1 cup or 237 ml) of water normally resting in the tray. Repeat at least once a month or as frequently as needed.

Use this water soluble tea tree oil disinfecting and mold control formula for bathroom and shower walls, curtains and doors. To make it first put 1 oz (2 tbsp, 30 ml) of glycerin in a container, then add 1/2 oz (1 tbsp, 15 ml) of pure tea tree oil. Seal and shake. Then add 1/2 oz (1 tbsp, 15 ml) of water. Tightly seal the container. Finally, shake the mixture vigorously. Use a sponge to apply this solution. Also good for disinfecting laundry.

Worst case condition – apply undiluted tea tree oil by putting a few drops onto a cotton swab, cotton ball or small paint brush and applying directly to the affected area. Repeat until condition improves and mold is gone.

Caution   If anyone has had a negative reaction to the tea tree oil, do not use it this way. The solution is to try another brand of tea tree oil. For more information refer to Chapter 3, Quality and Chemistry of Tea Tree Oil.

Plant Care

Fungus problems, molds, parasites and insect infestations are conditions tea tree oil can be used to treat with plants.

Research on the parasiticide and insecticide properties of tea tree oil with household variety plants is of an allegorical nature. Food producers and processors are testing tea tree oil solutions with fruits and vegetables for a variety of applications. The Melaleuca alternifolia tea tree is well protected by its own essential oils in the swampy humid conditions it generally grows in. In human parasite and insect infestations with lice, scabies, mosquitoes, etcetera, tea tree oil has generally proven itself to be safe, effective and non-toxic. The excellent antifungal properties of tree tree oil make it the perfect biological agent to combat fungal diseases.

I have successfully used it on rose bushes for mold and aphid infestations and on other household plants with problems. Tea tree oil is a much safer choice than many of the commercial products for plant care.

Recommendations

Fill a plant spray mister with 1 cup (8 oz, 237 ml) of distilled or cold boiled water and add 3-5 drops of tea tree oil, depending on the problem and hardiness of the plant. Shake vigorously. Mist the plant on the tops and bottoms of the foliage and the soil. Make sure to totally mist the affected area. You can leave it on the plant or wipe it off with a disposable paper towel. We prefer to leave it on. Repeat until condition is absent.

Put 10-20 drops in a room vaporizer or humidifier and let it permeate the air with tea tree oil vapors.

Worst case condition – apply pure tea tree oil by putting a few drops onto a cotton swab, cotton ball or small paint brush and applying directly to the affected area. Repeat daily, until plant shows signs of being restored to health, then use the spray mister.

Caution   If a plant starts to react negatively to the treatment discontinue applying pure tea tree oil or misting immediately. The longer the condition persists the longer it takes to help restore the plant to its natural healthy state.

If using tea tree oil to rid plants of parasites or insects, continue use for at least a week after infestation appears to be gone. Make sure the immediate area and other plants surrounding the affected one are also treated for the duration. This prevents a recurrence of the problem.

CHAPTER **10**

Pet Care Uses for
Cats, Dogs, Fish and Horses

Abscesses • Arthritis • Bites • Cuts • Dental Problems – Foul Breath, Gum Disease, Excessive Salivation • Dermatitis • Fish • Fleas • Joint and Muscular Disorders • Lice • Mange • Parasites • Puncture Wounds • Rashes • Ringworm • Sore Muscles • Sprains • Stings • Sunburns • Ticks • Vaccinations • Warts

Veterinary medicine is using tea tree oil for the treatment of cats, dogs, horses and other small pets. Undiluted pure tea tree oil, because of its concentration, can be irritating and generally should not be used on small animals, cats or dogs.

In September 1994 the *Small Animal Medicine and Surgery* veterinary journal reported that the National Animal Poison Control Center indicated *Melaleuca toxicosis,* when high doses of undiluted tea tree oil were topically applied to treat skin conditions in cats and dogs. Within 2 to 8 hours of use the following symptoms were noted: weakness, depression, poor coordination and muscle tremors. Within 3 to 4 days the reactions disappeared. Rarely, if ever should high doses of undiluted tea tree oil be used on pets. When recommended to treat difficult conditions, use sparingly with care and avoid the eye area. Watch your pet for any adverse reaction. If one occurs stop treatment with undiluted tea tree oil immediately. Generally a 15% tea tree oil dilution is preferred and is usually just as effective as pure tea tree oil.

This is the basis for a 15% tea tree oil dilution. As a base use 1 tsp (1/6 oz, 5 ml) of a non-allergenic fragrance free cream, gel, glycerin, lotion or cold pressed light vegetable oil and add 15-18 drops of pure tea tree oil to it. For a larger amount use 1 tbsp (1/2 oz, 15 ml) of the carrier base and add 45-54 drops of pure tea tree oil to it. Mix well before applying. Store in a glass or clear plastic container you can tightly seal and put in a cool place out of the sunlight. Label bottle: *Pet Care 15% Tea Tree Oil Mixture*.

Sources for herbal products containing tea tree oil include health food stores, pet stores and a consumer direct marketing group.

These guidelines are of a general nature based on the available information and suggestions of pet owners.

Abscesses

An abscess is due to an infection of a sebaceous gland. This results in an inflammation of the skin and localized painful swelling.

Recommendations

Clean the abscessed area with mild soap and warm water. Tea tree oil is an excellent antiseptic wound cleanser, analgesic (pain-killer) and it dissolves pus. Apply 1-2 drops of pure tea tree oil onto the abscess. When an abscess is draining make sure to clean area and keep applying pure tea tree oil 2-3 times a day, until redness disappears and a scab forms.

For hard-to-reach areas mix 8-12 drops of pure tea tree oil with 1 cup (8 oz, 237 ml) of water in a spray bottle. You can increase the amount of tea tree oil in the water if this dilution does not do the job. The nature of the abscess and size and sensitivity of the pet to tea tree oil are the determining factors. Shake contents vigorously before spraying.

Arthritis

Arthritis is an inflammation and/or pain in a joint or joints. Symptoms include swelling, redness of the skin and impaired motion. Two types of arthritis are: Osteoarthritis which is chronic, involves joints, especially those that are weight-bearing. Rheumatoid arthritis is chronic and manifested by inflammatory changes in joints which can be crippling. It is a degenerative joint disease.

Recommendations

Massage a soothing 2 1/2% tea tree oil dilution into the area. As a base use 1 tsp (1/6 oz, 5 ml) of a cold pressed light vegetable oil such as sweet almond or corn oil, or a cream and add 2-3 drops of pure tea tree oil. If you plan to frequently massage the area, use 1 tbsp (1/2 oz, 15 ml) of light vegetable oil or cream and add 6-9 drops of pure tea tree oil to it. Shake before each application.

When using magnetic wraps, first apply the 2 1/2% mixture onto the area. Wrap area in a clear plastic wrap. Then use the magnetic wrap according to its directions. With heating pads to prevent burns to the skin, make sure the pads temperature is set on low when using this tea tree oil mixture.

Bites

To prevent infection and ease the pain, tea tree oil is an excellent choice.

Recommendations

For extreme cases with dogs, put pure tea tree oil on a cotton ball and dab onto the affected area 2-3 times a day. Use sparingly, with care and avoid the eye area. Watch your pet for any adverse reaction. If one occurs stop treatment with undiluted tea tree oil immediately. Wait for symptoms to clear. Try the following 15% tea tree oil mixture.

For cats and small pets, use a 15% tea tree oil dilution in the area. As a base use 1 tsp (1/6 oz, 5 ml) of cold-pressed olive, sweet almond or corn oil and add 18 drops of pure tea tree oil. If you plan to frequently treat the area use 1 tbsp (1/2 oz, 15 ml) of cold-pressed oil and add 54 drops of pure tea tree oil to it. Mix well before applying. Put the 15% mixture on a cotton ball and dab onto the affected area 2-3 times a day.

Cuts – see Bites in this chapter

Dental Problems – Abscesses, Foul Breath, Gum Disease,
Excessive Salivation

Tea tree oil helps prevent infection, relieves inflammation and the pain of abscesses in the mouth, kills bacteria that causes plaque build up or foul breath, deals with problems causing excessive salivation, for a tooth that is removed or decayed it prevents infection and promotes healing. Its numerous properties are very beneficial for dealing with problems related to the mouth.

Recommendations

Use a squirt or spray bottle. To 1 tbsp (1/2 oz, 15 ml) glycerin add 9-10 drops of pure tea tree oil to make a water soluble mixture. Mix well. If a film of oil appears, it is not fully dissolved. Add a little more glycerin to the mixture, and shake the bottle again. When the mixture is cloudy the oil is evenly dispersed in it. Mix it with 1/2 cup (4 oz, 120 ml) of water in the squirt or spray bottle. Shake the bottle vigorously before each use and spray the affected area many times each day.

Once a week dip a toothbrush into this mixture and brush the teeth. This reduces the amount of bacteria in the mouth.

Dermatitis

Dermatitis is an inflammation of the skin. Characteristics may include flaky skin, redness, itchiness and rashes resulting in blisters, sores and scabs.

Recommendations

Make sure to monitor your pets condition by isolating it in a clean and dry pet carrier or cage to prevent any contagious conditions from spreading.

For dogs, first cut off the hair in and around the affected area. Then bathe your pet with water and mild soap. Massage 1-2 drops of pure tea tree oil into the location, 2-3 times a day, until the problem improves. Watch your pet for any adverse reaction. If one occurs stop treatment with undiluted tea tree oil immediately. Wait for symptoms to clear. The following 15% tea tree oil mixture is usually as effective as pure tea tree oil.

For cats and small pets, first cut off the hair in and around the affected area, then bathe pet with water and a mild soap. Then massage this 15% tea tree oil mixture into the area. As a base use 1 tsp (1/6 oz, 5 ml) of a non-allergenic fragrance free cream and add 15 drops of pure tea tree oil. If you plan to frequently treat the area use 1 tbsp (1/2 oz, 15 ml) of cream and add 45 drops of pure tea tree oil to it. Mix well before applying. Massage into the area 2-3 times a day.

Fish

For fungal diseases affecting fish in a tank or fish pond put 1-2 drops of pure tea tree oil in the water every day, for a period of a week. The amount varies depending on the size of the tank, or fish pond.

Fleas

Prevention

Fleas cause problems. Dogs sometimes chew the infested spots on their skin making them raw. Both dogs and cats can become infected with roundworm or tapeworms.

For regular bathing, wash the animal in a commercially prepared tea tree oil pet shampoo or add 3-4 drops of pure tea tree oil for each oz of the regular pet shampoo you use. Shake bottle vigorously, before each use. If it is a 10 oz bottle of shampoo, you add 30-40 drops of pure tea tree oil. You can occasionally use the 3-5% tea tree oil shampoo in this section.

Use tea tree oil as a flea, parasite and tick repellent. In a spray bottle blend 1 tsp (1/6 oz, 5 ml) of pure tea tree oil with 1 tbsp (1/2 oz, 15 ml) of a bay rum tincture, which is an alcohol extract. It makes the mixture water soluble and gives it a nice fragrance. Mix well. If a film of oil appears then the tea tree oil is not fully dissolved. Add a little more bay rum tincture to the mixture, and shake the bottle again. Add this to 1 cup (8 oz, 237 ml) of water. Shake vigorously before each application. Use mixture to keep their bedding and pet carriers free from pests. To repel insects spray your cat or dog before it goes outside.

Note that other essential oil combinations have been found to be helpful in dealing with fleas and ticks. Finding an effective tick repellent is very important, because of Rocky Mountain spotted fever and Lyme disease. Other essential oils that are good repellents include rose geranium, citronella oil, lemon, rosemary and California laurel. Some have adverse reactions, for example essential oil of lemon gets rid of fleas, but is also highly toxic to cats. Be sure to check the aromatherapy books recommended in the resources and bibliography sections at the back of this book.

During a flea infestation

Animals should be bathed daily during flea infestations. To avoid getting fleas in your house it is wise to do either of these choices outdoors.

Make a 3-4% tea tree oil pet shampoo. Blend 36-48 drops of pure tea tree oil, with 1/4 cup (2 oz, 60 ml) of the regular pet shampoo you use. Shake bottle vigorously, then use daily. Leave lather on for 3-5 minutes, then rinse. To improve the condition of the coat and prevent fleas, after and between washes sprinkle a moist sponge with 10-20 drops of pure tea tree oil and wipe their coat.

First wash with a mild pet shampoo and water. Hot spots should be clipped and treated with this mixture: In a spray mister blend 1 tbsp (1/3 oz, 15 ml) of pure tea tree oil, with 1 cup (8 oz, 237 ml) of water. Shake bottle vigorously, then thoroughly spray the animal down. Wait a 3-5 minutes. Treat the raw areas by taking a cotton ball, saturated with pure tea tree oil and dabbing the areas with it.

Joint and Muscular Disorders

Massage a soothing 2 1/2% tea tree oil mixture into the area. As a base use 1 tsp (1/6 oz, 5 ml) of a cold pressed light vegetable oil such as sweet almond or corn oil and add 3 drops of pure tea tree oil. If you plan to frequently massage the area use 1 tbsp (1/2 oz, 15 ml) of light vegetable oil and add 9 drops of pure tea tree oil to it. Shake before each application.

When using magnetic wraps, first apply the 2 1/2% mixture into the area. Wrap the area in a clear plastic wrap. Then use the magnetic wrap according to its directions.

With heating pads to prevent burns to the skin, make sure the pads temperature is set on low when using this tea tree oil mixture.

Lice

Lice are small wingless parasites that use humans and animals as a feeding source.

Recommendations

Wash animal with a gentle soap and water. Remove excess hair by clipping or shaving it off. Use a spray bottle to saturate the affected area with a combination of tea tree oil and water. Mix 15-20 drops of pure tea tree oil with 1 cup (8 oz, 237 ml) of water. When using a spray bottle shake vigorously before each application. Let it stand for 10-15 minutes, then dry the pet with a disposable paper towel. Throw out the paper towel. Do not use it for anything else.

For stubborn lice infested areas saturate a cotton ball with pure tea tree oil and apply it to the area. Do this for a period of at least a week, 2 times daily or until the lice are gone.

Isolate the pet. Disinfect pet carrier or kennel frequently by adding a few drops of pure tea tree oil to a cotton ball, damp disposable paper towel or use the following solution with a spray bottle or disposable paper towel. Mix 1 tsp (1/6 oz, 5 ml) of pure tea tree oil with 1/3 cup (2 2/3 oz, 79 ml) of water. For a larger amount mix 1 tbsp (1/2 oz, 15 ml) of pure tea tree oil to 1 cup (8 oz, 237 ml) of water. Shake vigorously before each application. If using a disposable paper towel or cotton ball, mix the solution thoroughly before each use. When using a spray bottle, shake vigorously before each application. Mist their bedding, sleeping area, pet carriers, kennel, etcetera.

Mange

Mange is a skin disease of mammals that causes itching, hair loss, etcetera. This condition is a difficult one to get rid of. Ask your veterinarian to give you additional suggestions for dealing with it.

Recommendations

Wash animal with a gentle soap and water. Remove excess hair by clipping or shaving it off. Use a spray bottle to saturate the affected area with the following mixture of tea tree oil and water. Mix 1 tsp (1/6 oz, 5 ml) of pure tea tree oil with 1/3 cup (2 2/3 oz, 79 ml) of water. For a larger amount 1 tbsp (1/2 oz, 15 ml) of pure tea tree oil to 1 cup (8 oz, 237 ml) of water. When using a spray bottle shake it vigorously before each application. Saturate the area with this mixture and let it stand for 10-15 minutes. Then dry the pet with a disposable paper towel. Throw out paper towel. Do not use it for anything else.

For stubborn areas saturate a cotton ball or disposable paper towel with pure tea tree oil and apply to the area. Do this 2 times daily, for a period of at least a week or until signs of mange are gone.

Isolate the pet. Disinfect pet carrier or kennel frequently by adding a few drops of pure tea tree oil to a cotton ball, damp disposable paper towel or use the following solution with a spray bottle or disposable paper towel. Mix 1 tsp (1/6 oz, 5 ml) of pure tea tree oil with 1/3 cup (2 2/3 oz, 79 ml) of water. For a larger amount mix 1 tbsp (1/2 oz, 15 ml) of pure tea tree oil to 1 cup (8 oz, 237 ml) of water. Shake vigorously before each application. If using a disposable paper towel or cotton ball, mix the solution thoroughly before each use. When using a spray bottle, shake vigorously before each application. Mist their bedding, sleeping area, pet carriers, kennel, etcetera.

Mouth Ulcers

Mouth ulcers are caused by a minor viral infection. The tiny blisters burst and form ulcers approximately 1/50th to 1/4 of an inch in diameter (2-10 mm) on or under the tongue, or on the inside of the pet's cheeks.

Recommendation

For mouth ulcers mix 8-12 drops of pure tea tree oil with 1 cup (8 oz, 237 ml) of water in a spray bottle. If this dilution does not do the job you can increase the amount of tea tree oil in the water. The nature of the mouth ulcer and size and sensitivity of the pet to tea tree oil, are the determining factors as to the concentration used. Shake contents vigorously before spraying.

Parasites

A parasite is an organism that lives on or in another living organism, without giving it something of value in return.

Use tea tree oil as a parasite, flea and tick repellent. In a spray bottle mix 1 tsp (1/6 oz, 5 ml) of pure tea tree oil and 1 cup (8 oz, 237 ml) of water. Shake vigorously before each application. Use mixture to keep their bedding, kennel and pet carriers free from pests. To repel insects spray your cat or dog before it goes outside.

Puncture Wounds

For puncture wounds it is important to clean the wound, prevent infection, reduce swelling and ease the pain.

Recommendations

Clean the puncture wound and area with mild soap and warm water. Tea tree oil is an excellent wound cleanser, pain-killer and anti-inflammatory. Apply 1-2 drops of pure tea tree oil onto the puncture wound and area. When a wound becomes infected, it is important when it is draining to make sure to clean the area and keep applying pure tea tree oil 2-3 times a day, until redness and infection disappear and a scab forms.

For hard-to-reach areas mix 8-12 drops of pure tea tree oil, with 1 cup (8 oz, 237 ml) of water in a spray bottle. You can increase the amount of tea tree oil in water, if this dilution does not do the job. The nature of the wound, size and sensitivity of the pet to tea tree oil, are the determining factors for how much tea tree oil you use. Shake contents of the bottle vigorously before spraying. Apply 2-3 times a day.

Rashes

A rash is an eruption of spots on the skin. Soothing and helping it to heal, prevents the pet from irritating the rash more and making it into an open sore, susceptible to infection.

Recommendations

For smaller rashes apply pure tea tree oil to the area. For larger rashes use a 2 1/2% tea tree oil solution in a light vegetable carrier base oil or cream. As a base use 1 tsp (5 ml) of a light vegetable oil such as sweet almond or corn oil, or a good hand cream or skin lotion and add 3 drops of pure tea tree oil. If you plan to frequently massage the rash use 1 tbsp (15 ml) of light vegetable oil or cream and 9 drops of pure tea tree oil. Shake or stir before each application.

Ringworm

Ringworm is a contagious skin disease caused by a fungus. It is evidenced by a scaly, red, O-shaped lesion that looks like the rings of Saturn. Common in dogs, cats and humans, it is easily transmitted.

Recommendations

First clip off the hair from the area affected with ringworm. Scrub with a mild soap and warm water.

Use a cotton ball to apply pure tea tree oil or a 5% tea tree oil mixture to the area. For a 5% dilution blend 1 tbsp (1/2 oz, 15 ml) of aloe vera gel or cold-pressed light vegetable oil (olive, sweet almond or corn) and 15 drops of pure tea tree oil. For a larger amount blend 1/4 cup (2 oz, 60 ml) of aloe vera gel or oil and 60 drops of pure tea tree oil. Repeat 2-3 times daily for one week or longer. Be patient, ringworm can take a while to clear up.

When washing pets, use a tea tree oil shampoo. Use a 2-4% commercially prepared tea tree oil pet shampoo or make your own. Add 20 drops (1/5 tsp, 1/30 oz, 1 ml) of tea tree oil for each oz (2 tbsp, 30 ml) of pet shampoo. Here's an example for a larger volume: Add 80 drops (4/5 tsp, 4 ml) of tea tree oil to 1/2 cup (4 oz, 118 ml) of shampoo. Shake vigorously before each use.

Disinfect bedding, pet carriers, kennel, etcetera by adding a few drops of pure tea tree oil to the wash water or use this: mix 15-20 drops of pure tea tree oil with 1 cup (8 oz, 237 ml) of water. Shake vigorously before each application. If using a sponge to apply the water and tea tree oil mixture, mix it thoroughly before using it. When using a spray bottle shake it vigorously before each application. Mist their bedding, sleeping area, pet carriers, etcetera.

Sore Muscles – see Sprains

Sprains

Massage a soothing 2 1/2% mixture into the area. As a base use 1 tsp (1/6 oz, 5 ml) of a cold pressed light vegetable oil (sweet almond or corn oil) or cream and add 3 drops of pure tea tree oil. If you plan to frequently massage the area use 1 tbsp (1/2 oz, 15 ml) of light vegetable oil or cream and add 9 drops of pure tea tree oil to it. Shake before each application.

When using magnetic wraps, first apply the 2 1/2% mixture into the area. Wrap the area in a clear plastic wrap. Then use the magnetic wrap, according to its directions.

With heating pads, to prevent burns to the skin, make sure the pads temperature is set on low when using this tea tree oil mixture.

Stings

For dogs, put pure tea tree oil on a cotton ball and dab onto the affected area 2-3 times a day.

For cats and small pets, use a 15% tea tree oil mixture in the area. As a base use 1 tsp (1/6 oz, 5 ml) of cold-pressed olive, sweet almond or corn oil and add 18 drops of pure tea tree oil. If you plan to frequently treat the area use 1 tbsp (1/2 oz, 15 ml) of cold-pressed oil and add 54 drops of pure tea tree oil to it. Mix well before applying. Put the 15%t mixture on a cotton ball and dab onto the affected area 2-3 times a day.

Sunburns

It is important to keep the area moist. For cats and dogs, mix equal amounts of pure tea tree oil and wheat germ or vitamin E oil. Apply at night. Do not expose the pet to the sun.

Ticks

Ticks are wingless, bloodsucking insects. These parasites infest humans and animals — cats, cows, dogs, horses, sheep, etcetera.

Prevention

Use tea tree oil as a flea, parasite and tick repellent. In a spray bottle mix 1 tsp (1/6 oz, 5 ml) of pure tea tree oil and 1 cup (8 oz, 237 ml) of water. Shake vigorously before each application. Unfortunately, the tea tree oil does not dissolve in this mixture and constant mixing is required. A better formula is just below. Use the mixture to keep their bedding and pet carriers free from pests. To repel insects spray your cat or dog before it goes outside.

This tea tree oil repellent mixture for ticks, fleas and parasite dissolves better in water and stays more evenly dispersed in the solution. In a spray bottle blend 1 tsp (1/6 oz, 5 ml) of pure tea tree oil with 1 tbsp (1/2 oz, 15 ml) of a bay rum tincture, which is an alcohol extract. It makes the mixture water soluble and gives it a nice fragrance. Mix well. If a film of oil appears, it is not fully dissolved. Add a little more bay rum tincture to the mixture, and shake bottle again. Add this to 1 cup (8 oz, 237 ml) of water. Shake vigorously before each application. Use this mixture to keep their bedding and pet carriers free from pests. To repel insects spray the cat or dog before it goes outside.

Note that other essential oil combinations have been found to be helpful in dealing with ticks. Finding an effective tick repellent is very important, because of Rocky Mountain spotted fever and Lyme disease. Other essential oils that are good repellents, include rose geranium, citronella oil, lemon, rosemary and California laurel. Some have adverse reactions, for example essential oil of lemon gets rid of fleas, but is also highly toxic to cats. Be sure to check the aromatherapy books recommended in the resources and bibliography sections at the back of this book.

Recommendation

Apply a drop of pure tea tree oil on the tick. Wait a few minutes, then remove with tweezers. The trick when using tweezers is to pull for a few or more seconds, then twist and pull, so the head comes out also. Continue putting and rubbing pure tea tree oil on the tick bites, 2-3 times a day, until they heal. This reduces swelling and the chance of infection.

Watch your pet for any adverse reaction. If one occurs stop treatment with undiluted tea tree oil immediately. Wait for symptoms to clear. Then try the following 15% tea tree oil mixture.

Use this 15% tea tree oil dilution on the tick bites. As a base use 1 tsp (1/6 oz, 5 ml) of a non-allergenic fragrance free cream and add 15 drops of pure tea tree oil. If you plan to frequently treat the area use 1 tbsp (1/2 oz, 15 ml) of cream and add 45 drops of pure tea tree oil to it. Mix well before applying. Massage into the area 2-3 times a day.

Vaccinations

For dogs, put pure tea tree oil on a cotton ball and dab onto the affected area 2-3 times a day.

For cats and small pets, put a 15% tea tree oil mixture on a cotton ball and dab onto the affected area. As a base use 1 tsp (1/6 oz, 5 ml) of cold-pressed olive, sweet almond or corn oil and add 18 drops of pure tea tree oil. Mix well before applying. Apply onto the affected area 2-3 times a day.

Warts

Warts are small, usually hard, tumorous growths on the skin, caused by a virus. Moisture helps them live. To soothe the pain of bleeding or itching due to warts, apply 1-2 drops of pure tea tree oil to the warts. Keep the area dry. Watch your pet for any adverse reaction. If one occurs stop treatment with undiluted tea tree oil immediately. Be patient, it can take weeks for the warts to disappear.

Congratulations! You have discovered the incredible powers and many uses of *Melaleuca alternifolia* – tea tree oil! Please share with us other ways you have successfully used this essential oil.

Personal Notes

Personal Notes

Personal Notes

Personal Notes

Appendix A
<u>Glossary of Terms</u>

Abscess – is due to an infection of a sebaceous gland. This results in an inflammation of the skin and localized painful swelling.

Alcohols – are pungent colorless liquids, forming esters in reaction with organic acids, sometimes used as a solvent when extracting essential oils or as a carrier base for essential oils.

Analgesic – pain relieving without affecting consciousness.

Aromatherapy – the practice and art of using the essential oils derived from plants, for healing purposes.

Aromatic baths – baths in which oils are used for cosmetic or healing purposes.

Arthritis – an inflammation and/or pain in a joint or joints. Symptoms include swelling, redness of the skin and impaired motion. Two types of arthritis are: Osteoarthritis which is chronic, involves joints, especially those that are weight-bearing. Rheumatoid arthritis is chronic and manifested by inflammatory changes in joints which can be crippling. It is a degenerative joint disease.

Astringent – that which contracts blood vessels and body tissues, reducing blood flow or having a biting or harsh quality.

Athlete's foot – is a contagious disease skin disease caused by a fungus, *Tinea pedis*, of the foot. It is commonly characterized by red, flaky or soggy skin and itching between the toes. The heels and soles can become covered in a white scaly skin. The fungus can also affect fingers and nails. Usually the affected skin cracks and becomes painful.

Bactericide – an agent that kills germs or bacteria.

Base oil – the main, essential or principal ingredient, acting as the vehicle for an essential oil. For therapeutic uses, such as aromatherapy, usually odorless high quality cold-pressed light vegetable oils are used.

Boil – a boil is technically called a *'furuncle'*. It is due to an infection of a sebaceous gland. This results in an inflammation of the skin and localized painful swelling.

Candida albicans – is also know as moniliasis or candidiasis, which can show itself in many forms. Candida albicans is a fungi which an excess of causes a yeast-like fungal infection. It thrives in the warm moist parts of the body such as the mouth (*candidiasis*), penis (*balanitis*), vagina (*thrush*), beneath the breasts and between folds of the buttock (*diaper rash*). Each condition manifests itself in a slightly different way, yet all are caused by the Candida albicans fungi.

Carbuncles – a collective mass of boils caused by the staphylococcus aureaus. Characterized by a painful node, covered with tight red skin that later thins and discharges pus. Commonly found on buttocks, upper back and nape of the neck. Extensive sloughing of the skin occurs when it is healing.

Carrier oil – see Base oil

Catarrh – is an inflammation of a mucous membrane. especially one chronically affecting the nose and air passages.

Chickenpox – is an acute, highly contagious viral disease, especially during childhood. It is caused by the *herpes zoster* virus, the same one responsible for shingles.It is characterized by skin eruptions of itchy spots, that blister, then turn to crusts. Also called Shingles or Zona.

Chiggers – are the tiny red larva of certain mites, whose bite causes severe itching.

Chilblains – is a painful swelling or sore, especially on the fingers or toes, caused by exposure to the cold or poor circulation.

Cold-pressed – mechanical method of extracting oil, by crushing the whole plant or part of the plant, without using heat. The oil is then filtered. This produces "virgin" oil.

Cold sore – is a viral infection, brought on by the herpes simplex type 1 virus, causing inflammation to the skin, usually the lips, mouth and face. It is characterized by small blisters. Herpes simplex type 1 is highly infectious and can spread to other parts of the body.

Colloidal – is a description used for a substance made up of small particles, insoluble, nondiffusible particles that remain suspended in a different type of medium, such as water, alcohol, etcetera.

Compress – a pad folded cloth pad, often moist or medicated that is applied to part of the body for healing, pressure , or to change the temperature, either up or down, of the area.

Corn – is an area of thickened hard skin between or on the toes. Sometimes it forms an inverted pyramid, which causes pressure in deeper layers of skin, resulting in pain.

Crabs – a lice infestation of the pubic hairs.

Cradle Cap – is a form of dermatitis newborn and very young babies exhibit. This unsightly scalp condition is thick yellowish crust lesions which develop on the scalp, face and sometimes extend to a scaling behind the ears.

Cuticles – are the hardened layer of outside skin, at the base and sides of a fingernail.

Cystitis – is a bladder infection caused by bacteria, that results in an inflammation of the bladder.

Dandruff – is a condition affecting the scalp. Overactive sebaceous gland secretions in the scalp cause scales to form, which may itch and burn. It may be caused by poor diet, inadequate stimulation of the scalp, poor blood circulation, pityrosporum ovale yeast which lives on the scalp, trichoplyton spp fungi, stress or chemical hair preparations.

Decongestant – a medication or treatment the relieves congestion, especially in the nose.

Dermatitis – is an inflammation of the skin. Characteristics may include flaky skin, redness, itchiness and rashes resulting in blisters, sores and scabs.

Diffuser – an apparatus that spreads out an essential oil, in the air, throughout a room.

Distillation – a process of heating a mixture, using steam and high pressure to separate the components of the mixture, and condensing the resulting vapors, to produce a concentrated purer essential oil.

Eczema – is a skin disorder characterized by inflammation, itching and scaliness.

Emollient – something that when applied to skin, soothes or softens it.

Emphysema – is a condition of the lungs, in which the air sacs become distended and lose elasticity.

Expectorant – a medicine or agent that helps to bring up phlegm or mucous, so it is expelled from the respiratory tract.

Extra-virgin – used to describe the highest quality grade of olive oil from the first pressing of the olives.

Fever – is an abnormally increased body temperature, which is a vital part of your bodies defense mechanism.

Flu – is an acute, contagious viral disease, characterized by inflammation of the respiratory tract, fever and muscular pain. It is also known as 'influenza'.

Fungal Infections of the skin – Fungal organisms are found on all healthy skin of humans, cats and dogs. It occurs when the natural balance is disturbed. In humans, by taking advantage of a persons weakened immune system, infections by opportunistic fungi become present. Examples of common one's include *Tinea pedis* (see Athlete's Foot), *Tinea cruris* (see Dhobi Itch and Jock Itch), *Tinea ungium* (see Ringworm), *Tinea capitis* (see Ringworm), *Tinea corporis* (see Ringworm).

Fungicidal – that which checks the growth of fungi, molds or spores.

Furuncle – is the technical term for '*boil*'. see Boil

Gingivitis – is a build up of bacterial plaque, that causes the gums to swell, redden and bleed easily.

Halitosis – is bad smelling breath.

Hemorrhoid – is a painful swelling of a vein, in the region of the anus or rectum, often with bleeding. It is a varicose vein. Also known as Pile(s)

Hives – are an allergic skin condition or hypersensitive reaction characterized by itching, burning and the formation of smooth patches.

Impetigo – is an highly contagious skin disease with eruptions of pustules, pus filled blisters or pimples. The infection mainly affects children. It is usually caused by the *streptococcus* or *staphylococcus bacteria*. The appearance of spots or inflamed patches is normally seen on the scalp, neck and face. Sometimes blisters that crust over, appear on the knees and hands.

Influenza – commonly known as flu, is an acute, contagious viral disease, characterized by inflammation of the respiratory tract, fever and muscular pain.

Inhalation – to breath in a vapor, using the lungs and respiratory system as the delivery system for the essential oil into the blood stream.

Leg ulcer – is an open sore on the leg, discharging pus.

Leucorrhoea – is an inflammation of the vagina that is caused by an excessive amount of bacteria or fungi. Often there is a thick yellow or white discharge accompanied by severe itching to the vagina.

Lipophilic – means fat loving.

Nasal Ulcer – is an open sore in the nose, discharging pus.

Meningitis – an inflammation of the three membranes that envelop the brain and spinal column.

Miscible — to mix, or can be mixed.

Paronychia — is a fungal infection that affects toenails and fingernails. Cuticles become painful and red, with a small discharge. Skin below nails becomes discolored.

Piles — see Hemorrhoids

Plantar Wart — are small, usually less than 1/4 inch, sometimes larger. They are caused by a virus invasion through an abrasion or microscopic cut on the sole of the foot. The warts grow inward and under the skin. The pressure exerted by walking causes the area to become flattened until it becomes callused. The location has a tiny black on on the surface. They can be very painful. They are difficult to get rid of and may reappear.

Poison Ivy — is a plant having leaves of three leaflets and ivory-colored berries. When the sap from the plant comes in contact with the skin, it causes a severe rash, redness, swelling, blistering, and intense itching in sensitive people.

Poison Oak — is a climbing vine, related to poison ivy.

Prickly heat — is a skin eruption caused by inflammation of the sweat glands.

Pruritis — or itching is a most irritating condition, generally accompanying a mild vaginal infection, such as cervicitis or trichomonal vaginitis.

Psoriasis — is a chronic skin disease, characterized by scaly, reddish patches and itching. The inflammation sometimes shows up as silvery scales that appear on elbows, knees, scalp and torso. It is not contagious. The cause is generally unknown.

Rash — an eruption of spots on the skin.

Ringworm — is a contagious skin disease caused by a fungus. It is evidenced by a scaly, red, O-shaped lesion that looks like the rings of Saturn. Common in dogs, cats and humans, it is easily transmitted.

Salpingitis – is caused by the streptococci and staphylococci bacteria. It is an inflammation of the Fallopian tubs. Symptoms can include fever, vaginal discharge and vomiting.

Scabies – is a highly contagious, itching skin disease caused by the itch mite, *sarcoptes scabiei.* The female mite burrows under the skin to lay its eggs. The newly hatched mites burrow out of the skin and this causes severe itching and irritation. Possible signs include small red pimples and scratching, which may result in sores, that can become infected. Secondary infections are of great concern with scabies. Easily transmitted from person to person. Area's commonly affected by this condition include the groin, penis, nipples and skin between the fingers. Disinfect bed linens, mattress and clothing to prevent reinfection.

Shingles – is the nontechnical term used for the *herpes zoster virus*, the same one responsible for chickenpox.

Sinusitis – is an inflammation of the sinuses. The mucous membranes that line the cavities above, behind and to each side of the nose become swelled.

Sitz bath – is a therapeutic bath in which only the hips and buttocks are immersed.

Stye – a small inflamed swelling on the rim of an eyelid.

Ticks – are wingless, bloodsucking insects. These parasites infest humans and animals – cows, sheep, etcetera...

Tinea – is a fungal infection, caused by a microscopic fungal mold.

Tropical Ulcer (Naga Sore) – A large painless sore develops, usually on the legs or feet, that becomes infected by bacteria. Happens in hot, humid climates.

Ulcers – are open sores on the skin or mucous membrane, that discharges pus.

Urethritis – a bacterial infection of the urethra which usually precedes an attack of cystitis.

Vaginitas – an inflammation of the canal from vulva to the uterus.

Vaporization – to change something into a steam suspension (vapor) or mist for dispersion through the air. The air is used a delivery system for an essential oil. It can be done by heating, spraying or evaporating an essential oil.

Varicose ulcers – are enlarged veins abnormally and irregularly swollen, that form on the lower legs, often as a result of varicose veins. The slightest break in the skin, can cause a sore or ulcer to develop that takes a long time to heal. The aged, usually suffering from poor circulation, are very prone to this condition.

Veruccae – see Warts

Virgin oil – highest quality vegetable oil extracted from the first pressing of the plant. Extra-virgin used to describe the highest grade of the first pressing of olive oil.

Warts – a small, usually hard, tumorous growth on the skin, caused by a virus.

Zona – is also called shingles, it is caused by the *herpes zoster virus*, the same one responsible for chickenpox.

Appendix B
Resources

U.S.A.
General Information and Natural Product Resources
American Botanical Council
P.O. Box 201660
Austin, TX 79720
(512) 331-8868 Fax (512) 231-1924
email: custserv@herbalgram.org
Resource center for herb research and regulations. Publishes
HerbalGram.

American Tea Tree Association (ATTA)
c/o AllerClean, Inc.
6400 Black Horse Pike
Egg Harbor Township, NJ 08234
Association monitors quality standards for imported tea tree
oil. Focus on getting FDA approval for tea tree oil as an effective and safe ingredient for various products.

Aroma Vera
5901 Rodeo Rd.
Los Angeles, CA 90016-4312
(800) 669-9514 Fax (310) 280-0395
Supplier of essential oil products for health and beauty
purposes.

Aura Cacia also known a Frontier Co-Operative Herbs
3021 78th Street
Norway, Iowa 42318
(800) 729-5422 Head Office
(800) 786-1388 Order Line
(800) 437-3301 Customer Service
Supplier of tea tree oil, herbal and other natural products.

Centers for Disease Control and Prevention
1600 Clifton Road NE
Atlanta, Georgia 30333
It is part of the department of Health and Prevention and
provides information to the public on specific diseases.

Consumer Product Safety Commission Chemical Hazards
Program
5401 Westbard Avenue
Washington, D.C. 20207
Regulates consumer products. Provides information on chemi-
cals, particularly those used in homes.

Food and Drug Administration
Freedom of Information Office
5600 Fishers Lane
Rockville, Maryland 20857
Responds to written requests for information on foods and
some questions on low level exposure to toxic chemicals.

Herb Pharm
20260 Williams Highway
Williams, OR 97544
(800) 348-4377 Fax (541) 846-6112

Herb Research Foundation
107 Pearl Street, Suite 200
Boulder, CO 80302
(303) 449-2265 Fax (303) 449-7849
Supplier of botanical research services. Co-publishes
HerbalGram with American Botanical Council.

U.S.A.
Tea Tree Oil Wholesale
<u>Mail Order and Retail Product Suppliers</u>

Australian Holdings Inc.
5855 Green Valley circle #102
Culver City, CA 90230
(310) 348-1993 Fax (310) 348-9074
Bulk sales supplier of tea tree oil.

The Body Shop by Mail
45 Horsehill Road
Cedar Knolls, NJ 07927-2014
(800) 426-3922
Supplier tea tree oil body care products.

Derma-E
9400 Lurline Avenue, #C-1
Chatsworth, CA 91311
(800) 521-3342 Fax (818) 718-6907
Supplier of tea tree oil hair and skin care products.

Dessert Essence and Tea Tree Solutions brand names
9510 Vassar Avenue, Unit A
Chatsworth, CA 91311
(800) 848-8331 Fax (818) 705-8525
Supplier of tea tree oil health and body care products.

Espial USA Ltd.
7045 South Fulton Street, Suite 200
Englewood, CO 80112
(800) 695-5555 Fax (303) 792-3933
Multi-level network marketing company that supplies personal
care products with tea tree oil.

Essential Care USA, Inc.
661 Palisade Avenue
Englewood Cliffs, NJ 07632
(201) 567-9004 Fax (201) 567-8853
Bulk oil supplier of tea tree oil and products for retail markets
- health and beauty aids.

Inside BestSeller Product and Information Services
1623 Military Rd., Suite 203
Niagara Falls, NY 14304-1745
(800) 595-1955 Fax (800) 458-0025
Supplier of tea tree oil, natural products and books.

International Sourcing Inc.
121 Pleasant Ave.
Upper Saddle river, NJ 07458
(201) 934-8900
Bulk order supplier of tea tree oil.

Jason Natural Products
8468 Warner Drive
Culver City, CA 90232
(310) 838-7543 Fax (310) 838-9274
email: jnp@jason-natural.com
Supplier of tea tree oil health and beauty products.

John Paul Mitchell Systems
26455 Golden Valley Road
Saugus, CA 91350
Order line (805) 298-0400
Head office (310) 248-3888
Supplier of tea tree oil body care products.

Marco Industries
3431 West Thunderbird, Suite 144
Phoenix, AZ 85023
(800) 726-1612
email: marco-lesi@juno.com
Supplier tea tree oil antiseptic herbal ointments, suppositories,
douche, toothpaste and other products.

Melaleuca Inc.
3910 S. Yellowstone Hwy
Idaho Falls, ID 83402
Consumer direct marketing company. Supplies personal care,
vitamins, natural products, plus over 60 products containing

tea tree oil for personal, health, pet and environmentally friendly home care products.
(208) 522-0700 Fax (208) 528-2090

Mitek Laboratories Inc.
102 Haverford Road
Pittsburgh, PA 15238-1620
(412) 967-9674 Fax (412) 963-7747
Bulk order sales of tea tree oil.

Rye Pharmaceuticals Pty. Ltd.
Beard Plaza
6540 Washington Street
Yountville, CA 94599
(707) 944-8090 Fax (707) 944-8092
email: ryemkt@msn.com
Supplier of tea tree oil products for burns in pump dispensers, tube and sterile burn blanket dressings.

Starwest Botanicals, Inc.
11253 Trade Center Drive
Rancho Cordova, CA 95742
(800) 800-4372 or (916) 638-8100 Fax (916) 638-8293
Supplier of tea tree oil only for wholesale customers.

Tea Tree Solutions see Dessert Essence in this section.

Thursday Plantation, Inc.
330 Carillo Street
Santa Barbara, CA 93101
(805) 566-0354 Fax (805) 566-9798
Order line (800) 645-9000
Supplier tea tree oil and products for wholesale and retail markets.

Water Jel Technologies
243 Veterans Blvd.
Carlstadt, NJ 07072
(201) 507-8300 Fax (201) 507-8325
Medical supplier tea tree oil burn blanket dressings.

Canada

Australian Bodycare of Canada, Ltd.
915 Esquimalt Avenue
West Vancouver, British Columbia V7T 1J9 Canada

Brueckner Group
4717 14th Avenue
Markham, Ontario L3R 3K3 Canada
(905) 479-2121 Fax (905) 479-2122
Supplier tea tree oil skin care products.

Inside BestSeller Product and Information Services
226 Queen Street South
Kincardine, Ontario N2Z 2S5 Canada
(800) 595-1955 Fax (800) 458-0025
Supplier of natural health products and books.

Melaleuca Canada Inc. (division of Melaleuca Inc. USA)
Canadian head office in Winnipeg, Manitoba
Consumer direct marketing company. Supplies personal care,
vitamins, natural products, plus over 60 products containing
tea tree oil for personal, health, pet and environmentally
friendly home care products.
(208) 522-0700 Fax (208) 528-2090

Natural Trading Ltd.
4454 West 10th Avenue
Vancouver, British Columbia V6R 2H9 Canada
Supplier for the United Kingdom's *Aqua Oleum* line of essential oils and tea tree oil products.

Purity Life Health Products, Ltd.
100 Elgin St., S.
Acton, Ontario L7J 2W1 Canada
(519) 853-3511 Fax (519) 853-4660
Canadian distributor for Thursday Plantation tea tree oil products.

Swiss Herbal Remedies, Ltd.
35 Leek Cres.
Richmond Hill, Ontario
(905) 886-9500 Fax (905) 886-5434
Supplies tea tree oil, herbal, vitamin, mineral and personal care products

Australia

The Australian Essential Oil Company Pty. Ltd.
575 Myall Creek Rd., Box 158
Bora Ridge, Coraki NSW 2471 Australia
(616) 683-2121 Fax (616) 683-2603
Supplier of bulk tea tree oil in the following grades: cosmetic, industrial, pharmaceutical, organic and technical.

Australian tea Tree Export and Marketing Company and Australian Tea Tree Industry Association (ATTA)
P. O. Box 20
Tweed Heads, NSW 2485 Australia
(616) 621-2221 Fax (616) 674-2475
Marketing and export sales cooperative venture of major producers of tea tree oil.

Australian Tea Tree Oil Research Institute (ATTORI)
Southern Cross university
Military Road
Lismore, NSW 248 Australia
(616) 622-3211 Fax (616) 622-3459
A major new tea tree oil research and product development facility. Main Camp Tree Oil Group is responsible for the facility. Research under the auspices of Southern Cross University, Lismore, Australia. Staff of scientists and researchers. Advisory board is a cross section of experts from therapeutic, pharmacological and research sciences.
Clinical studies will be conducted to verify claims from anecdotal information and 'in-vitro' (test tube) studies. Focus on

product licensing and manufacturing geared to making tea tree oil a mainstream therapeutic component as an essential oil and for use in products.

Bronson and Jacobs Pty. Ltd.
Parkview drive, Australia Centre
Homebush Bay NSW, 2140 Australia
(6129) 394-3288 Fax (6129) 394-3222
Grower and producer of tea tree oil for domestic and international markets.

Creatique Australia Pty. Ltd.
P.O. Box 2420
Fortitude Valley BC
Queensland 4006 Australia
(6173) 254-1851 Fax (6173) 254-1841
email: creatique@gil.com.au
Supplier of a complete range of natural personal care products, some using tea tree oil.

Essential Resources of Sydney, Australia
Essential Care USA, Inc. is a division of this company.
661 Palisade Avenue
Englewood Cliffs, NJ 07632
(201) 567-9004 Fax (201) 567-8853
Bulk oil supplier of tea tree oil and products for retail markets - health and beauty aids.

Eureka Oils Pty. Ltd.
Jonson Street
Bryon Bay NSW 2481 Australia
(616) 685-6333
Supplier of a bottled 20% tea tree oil water soluble mixture.

Gateway Pharmaceuticals
274 Pennant Hills Rd., Box 217
Thornleigh, NSW 2120 Australia
(612) 484-4764 Fax (612) 875-3731
Grower and supplier of tea tree oil in bulk, a well as in animal and veterinary disinfecting products.

G.R. Davis Pty. Ltd.
9 Apollo Street, Suite 3
Warriewood, NSW 2102 Australia
(6129) 979-9844 Fax (6129) 979-9608
Supplier of tea tee oil for Australian and export markets, for
their own plantation and other growers.

Macquarie Plantations Pty. Ltd.
17-7 Chapel Lane
Baulkiiam Hills NSW, 2153 Australia
(6129) 686-7891 Fax (6129) 639-7831
Co-operative research, development and supplier of bulk tea
tree oil for domestic and export sales.

Main Camp tea Tree Oil Group
85 Tamar street, Box 407
Ballina NSW, 2478 Australia
(616) 686-3099 Fax (616) 686-2722
Major supplier of the following grades of bulk tea tree oil:
International Standard Organization (ISO) and pharmaceutical
grades. Largest tea tree oil plantation.

Sunspirit Oils Pty. Ltd.
6 Ti-tree Place, Box 85
Byron Bay NSW, 2481 Australia
(616) 685-6333 Fax (616) 865-6313
Supplier and exporter of 25 ml bottles of pure tea tree oil and
50 gm tea tree oil ointment.

Thursday Plantation Laboratories Limited
Pacific Highway Ballina
NSW 2478 Australia
(02) 6886-7273 Fax (02) 6686-6485
International Fax +61-2-6686-7485
First commercial tea tree plantation of high quality medicinal
grade oil. Established in 1976. State of the art pharmacological
grade manufacturing, chemical and microbiological laboratory
facilities. Exports to 25 countries.

Appendix C
Conventional American Fluid Measurements
and
<u>Their Standard International Equivalents</u>

1 tsp	=	1/3 tbsp	=	1/6 oz	=	4.9 ml
3 tsp	=	1 tbsp	=	1/2 oz	=	14.8 ml
6 tsp	=	2 tbsp	=	1 oz	=	29.6 ml
1 oz	=	2 tbsp	=	0.0296 l	=	29.6 ml
1 c	=	16 tbsp	=	8 oz	=	236.6 ml
1 l	=	1.0567 qt	=	33.814 oz	=	4.2268 c
1 l	=	1000 ml	=	2.113 pt		
20 drops	=	1/30 oz	=	1 ml		

Pure Tea Tree Essential Oil
is measured in drops due to its high concentration.

tsp – teaspoon	tbsp – tablespoon	c – cup	pt – pint
oz – fluid ounce	qt – liquid quart	ml – milliliter	l – liter

Appendix D
References

1. Arthur Penfold and F. R. Morrison, 'Australian Tea Trees of Economic Value', *Technological Museum Bulletin*, vol. 14, 1929

2. M. Coutts, 'The Bronchoscopic Treatment of Bronchiectasis, *Medical Journal of Australia*, July 1937

3. Robert Goldsborough, 'Ti-Tree Oil', *The Manufacturing Chemist,* February, 1939, pp. 57, 58 and 60.

4. Ernest Guenther, 'Tea Tree Oils', *Soap and Sanitary Chemicals*, August/September, 1942

5. W.A. Poucher, 'Tea Tree Oil', *Perfumes, Cosmetics and Soap*, 4th ed., 1:370, 1936

6. Arthur Penfold & F.R. Morrison, 'Some Notes of the Essential Oil of Melaleuca Alternifolia', *Australian Journal of Pharmacy*, March 1937, pp 274

7. Henry Feinblatt, 'Cajeput - Type Oil for the Treatment of Furunculosis', *Journal of the National Medical Association*, vol.52:1, January 1960, pp. 32-34

8. Eduardo Pena, 'Melaleuca Alternifolia Oil: It Use for Trichomonal Vaginitis and Other Vaginal Infections', *Journal of Obstetrics and Gynecology* 19 (1962), p. 792-95.

9. M. Walker , 'Clinical Investigation of Australian Melaleuca alternifolia for a Variety of Common Foot Problems', *Current Pediatry* (April 1972)

10. M. F. Beylier, Perfumer and Flavourist, 4:23. April/May 1979, pp. 23-25

11. Paul Belaiche, 'Treatment of Skin Infection with the Essential Oil of *'Melaleuca Alternifolia'*, and 'Treatment of vaginal Infections of Candida albicans with the Essential Oil of *'Melaleuca Alternifolia'*, Phytotherapy 15 (1985)

12. R.C.S. Barnetson, *Australian Journal of Pharmacy,* " October (1990), vol. 153. pp 455-458

13. A.L. Blackwell, *Lancet* 337 (1991), p. 300

14. A. Shemesh and W.L. Mayo, 'Tea Tree Oil - natural antiseptic and fungicide', *International Journal of Alternative and Complementary Medicine* (Dec. 1991), p. 12.

15. Carson, Cookson, Farrelly and Rilley, 'Susceptibility of methicillin-resistant *Staphylococcus aureus* to the essential oil of Melaleuca alternifolia', *Journal of Antimicrobial Chemotherapy,* vol 35 pp. 421-424, 1995

16. Ryan, R., 'Oil of *Melaleuca alternifolia* Dissolved in Liquid Carbon Dioxide Propellant (Bactigas™) Used for the Control of Bacteria and Fungi in Air Conditioning Systems', *Modern Phytotherapy - the Clinical Significance of Tea Tree and Other Essential Oils,* vol. 2 of the proceedings of a two day conference at Macquarie University, Sydney, Dec. 1 & 2, 1990

17. Smith, Martha D., and Patricia L. Navilliat, "A new protocol for antimicrobial testing of oils", Journal of Microbiological Methods,28, pp. 21-24, 1997

18. A. de Groot and J. Weyland, vol. 27, no.4 (1992) Contact Dermatitis cited in *Natural Database U.K. Aromatherapy,* vol. 1, p. 22.

19. R. Tisserand, 'Athlete's Foot', International Journal of Aromatherapy 2.3 (1989), p. 19.

20. 'Ti-tree Oil and Chickenpox', *Aromatherapy Quarterly,* Summer 1986, p. 12

21. Altman, P. M., 'Summary of Safety Studies concerning Australian Tree Oil,' *Modern Phytotherapy - the Clinical Significance of Tea Tree and Other Essential Oils,* vol. 2 of the proceedings of a two day conference at Macquarie University, Sydney, Dec. 1 & 2, 1990

22. Barnes, B., 'The Vaginal Range of Formulations containing Tea Tree Oil', *Modern Phytotherapy - the Clinical Significance of Tea Tree and Other Essential Oils*, vol. 2 of the proceedings of a two day conference at Macquarie University, Sydney, Dec. 1 & 2, 1990

23. Barnes, B, 'The Development of Topical Applications containing Tea Tree Oil for Vaginal Conditions', *Modern Phytotherapy - the Clinical Significance of Tea Tree and Other Essential Oils*, vol. 1 of the proceedings of a two day conference at Macquarie University, Sydney, Dec. 1 & 2, 1990

23. Cabot, Dr. S, 'The Use of Tea Tree in Clinical Practice', *Modern Phytotherapy - the Clinical Significance of Tea Tree and Other Essential Oils*, vol. 1 of the proceedings of a two day conference at Macquarie University, Sydney, Dec. 1 & 2, 1990

24. Dean, C., 'The Marketing of Tea Tree Oil for its True Worth', *Modern Phytotherapy - the Clinical Significance of Tea Tree and Other Essential Oils*, vol. 2 of the proceedings of a two day conference at Macquarie University, Sydney, Dec. 1 & 2, 1990

25. Dean, C and P. Daffy, 'A Natural Answer to Acne Dilemma', *Modern Phytotherapy - the Clinical Significance of Tea Tree and Other Essential Oils*, vol. 2 of the proceedings of a two day conference at Macquarie University, Sydney, Dec. 1 & 2, 1990

26. Hellyer, Dr. O., 'Review of Current Safety Efficacy Studies on Melaleuca Oil to Approved Protocols', *Modern Phytotherapy - the Clinical Significance of Tea Tree and Other Essential Oils*, vol. 2 of the proceedings of a two day conference at Macquarie University, Sydney, Dec. 1 & 2, 1990

27. Home, V., 'Antimicrobial Activity in Perspective', *Modern Phytotherapy - the Clinical Significance of Tea Tree and Other Essential Oils*, vol. 2 of the proceedings of a two day conference at Macquarie University, Sydney, Dec. 1 & 2, 1990

28. Merkur, Dr. H., 'The Impact of Human Papilloma Virus (HPV) in Gynaecology', *Modern Phytotherapy - the Clinical Significance of Tea Tree and Other Essential Oils*, vol. 1 of the proceedings of a two day conference at Macquarie University, Sydney Dec. 1 & 2, 1990

29. Merry, K.A., 'Composition of Oils from *Melaleuca alternifolia, Melaleuca linariifolia, Melaleuca dissitisflora*. Implications for the Australian Standard, Oil of Melaleuca - Terpinen-4-ol Type', *Modern Phytotherapy - the Clinical Significance of Tea Tree and Other Essential Oils*, vol. 2 of the proceedings of a two day conference at Macquarie University, Sydney, Dec. 1 & 2, 1990

30. Sachs, Prof. R., '*Melaleuca alternifolia*: An Estimate of its Potential as a Crop for California', *Modern Phytotherapy - the Clinical Significance of Tea Tree and Other Essential Oils*, vol. 2 of the proceedings of a two day conference at Macquarie University, Sydney, Dec. 1 & 2, 1990

31. Setright, R., 'A Phytotherapeutic Approach to the Immune System and Viral Infections', *Modern Phytotherapy - the Clinical Significance of Tea Tree and Other Essential Oils*, vol. 1 of the proceedings of a two day conference at Macquarie University, Sydney, Dec. 1 & 2, 1990

32. Stewart, D., 'The Scientific Basis and Clinical Significance of Essential Oil Use in Phytotherapy', *Modern Phytotherapy - the Clinical Significance of Tea Tree and Other Essential Oils*, vol. 1 of the proceedings of a two day conference at Macquarie University, Sydney, Dec. 1 & 2, 1990

33. Williams, Dr. L., 'The Modern Tea Tree Oil Story', *Modern Phytotherapy - the Clinical Significance of Tea Tree and Other Essential Oils*, vol. 1 of the proceedings of a two day conference at Macquarie University, Sydney, Dec. 1 & 2, 1990

34. Williams, Dr. L., 'Selection and Breeding of Superior Strains of Melaleuca Species to Produce Low Cost, High Quality Tea Tree Oil', *Modern Phytotherapy - the Clinical Significance of Tea Tree and Other Essential Oils,* vol. 2 of the proceedings of a two day conference at Macquarie University, Sydney, Dec. 1 & 2, 1990

35. Fogarty, J., 'Clinical Investigation of a Tea Tree Oil Preparation for the Rehydration of the Skin in the Lower Limb', *Modern Phytotherapy - the Clinical Significance of Tea Tree and Other Essential Oils,* vol. 2 of the proceedings of a two day conference at Macquarie University, Sydney, Dec. 1 & 2, 1990

Bibliography

Altman, P. M., 'Summary of Safety Studies concerning Australian Tree Oil,' *Modern Phytotherapy - the Clinical Significance of Tea Tree and Other Essential Oils*, vol. 2 of the proceedings of a two day conference at Macquarie University, Sydney, Dec. 1 & 2, 1990

Baerheim Svendson, Scheffer, *Essential Oils and Aromatic Plants*, Dr. W. Junk, 1985

Barnes, B., 'The Vaginol Range of Formulations containing Tea Tree Oil', *Modern Phytotherapy - the Clinical Significance of Tea Tree and Other Essential Oils*, vol. 2 of the proceedings of a two day conference at Macquarie University, Sydney, Dec. 1 & 2, 1990

Barnes, B, 'The Development of Topical Applications containing Tea Tree Oil for Vaginal Conditions', *Modern Phytotherapy - the Clinical Significance of Tea Tree and Other Essential Oils*, vol. 1 of the proceedings of a two day conference at Macquarie University, Sydney, Dec. 1 & 2, 1990

Barnetson, R.C.S., *Australian Journal of Pharmacy*, " October (1990), vol. 153. pp 455-458

Barnes-Svarney, Patricia, *The New York Public library Science Desk Reference*, MacMillan, New York, New York, 1995

Belaiche, Paul, *Traits de Phyto-therapie et d'Aromatherapie*, 3 vols. Libraire Maloine, Paris, 1979.

Belaiche, Paul, 'Treatment of Skin Infection with the Essential Oil of *'Melaleuca Alternifolia'*, and 'Treatment of vaginal Infections of Candida albicans with the Essential Oil of *'Melaleuca Alternifolia'*, Phytotherapy 15, 1985

Bernadet, Marcel, *La Phyto-Aromatherapie Pratique*. Editions Dangles, St. Jean de Braye, 1983

Beylier, M. F., *Perfumer and Flavourist*, 4:23. April/May 1979, pp. 23-25

Blackwell, A.L., *Lancet* 337, p. 300, 1991

Bubny, Paul , *Consumer Education Series: Tea Tree Oil*, Health Foods Business magazine, U.S.A., July 1989

Cabot, Dr. S, 'The Use of Tea Tree in Clinical Practice', *Modern Phytotherapy - the Clinical Significance of Tea Tree and Other*

Essential Oils, vol. 1 of the proceedings of a two day conference at Macquarie University, Sydney, Dec. 1 & 2, 1990

Carson, Cookson, Farrelly and Rilley, 'Susceptibility of methicillin-resistant *Staphylococcus aureus* to the essential oil of Melaleuca alternifolia', *Journal of Antimicrobial Chemotherapy*, vol 35 pp. 421-424, 1995

Coutts, M., 'The Bronchoscopic Treatment of Bronchiectasis, *Medical Journal of Australia*, July 1937

Culpeper, *Complete Herbal*, W. Foulsham & Co., London, 1952

Dean, C., 'The Marketing of Tea Tree Oil for its True Worth', *Modern Phytotherapy - the Clinical Significance of Tea Tree and Other Essential Oils*, vol. 2 of the proceedings of a two day conference at Macquarie University, Sydney, Dec. 1 & 2, 1990

Dean, C and P. Daffy, 'A Natural Answer to Acne Dilemma', *Modern Phytotherapy - the Clinical Significance of Tea Tree and Other Essential Oils*, vol. 2 of the proceedings of a two day conference at Macquarie University, Sydney, Dec. 1 & 2, 1990

de Groot, A. and J. Weyland, vol. 27, no.4 (1992) Contact Dermatitis cited in *Natural Database U.K. Aromatherapy*, vol. 1, p. 22.

Drury, Susan, Tea Tree Oil: A Medicine Kit in a Bottle, C.W. Daniel Company, Ltd., Essex, England, 1991

Duraffourd, Paul, *The Best of Health: Thanks to Essential Oils*, Cevic, 1984

Feinblatt, Henry, 'Cajeput - Type Oil for the Treatment of Furunculosis', *Journal of the National Medical Association*, vol.52:1, January 1960, pp. 32-34

Fogarty, J., 'Clinical Investigation of a Tea Tree Oil Preparation for the Rehydration of the Skin in the Lower Limb', *Modern Phytotherapy - the Clinical Significance of Tea Tree and Other Essential Oils*, vol. 2 of the proceedings of a two day conference at Macquarie University, Sydney, Dec. 1 & 2, 1990

Foster, Stephen, 'Tea Tree and Its relatives: A Little medicine, a Little Marketing.' *The Herb Companion*, pp. 48-51, February/March,1994

Foster, Stephen, 'Why the To-Do about tea Tree Oil?', *Vegetarian Times*, pp. 98-101, October 1995

Goldsborough, Robert, 'Ti-Tree Oil', *The Manufacturing Chemist*, February, 1939, pp. 57, 58 and 60.

Guenther, Ernest, 'Tea Tree Oils', *Soap and Sanitary Chemicals*, August/September, 1942

Hellyer, Dr. O., 'Review of Current Safety Efficacy Studies on Melaleuca Oil to Approved Protocols', *Modern Phytotherapy - the Clinical Significance of Tea Tree and Other Essential Oils*, vol. 2 of the proceedings of a two day conference at Macquarie University, Sydney, Dec. 1 & 2, 1990

Home, V., 'Antimicrobial Activity in Perspective', *Modern Phytotherapy - the Clinical Significance of Tea Tree and Other Essential Oils*, vol. 2 of the proceedings of a two day conference at Macquarie University, Sydney, Dec. 1 & 2, 1990

Humphrey, E. M., 'A New Australian Germicide', *Medical Journal of Australia* 1, 1930

Ingram, Cass, *Killed on Contact: The Tea Tree Oil Story, Nature's Finest Antiseptic*, Literary Visions Publishing, Cedar Rapids, Iowa, 1992

Lawless, Julia, *The Encyclopedia of Essential Oils*, Element Inc., Rockport, Massachusetts, 1992

Lee, William H. and Lynn Lee, *The Book of Practical Aromatherapy*, Keats Publishing, New Canaan, Connecticut 1992.

Merkur, Dr. H., 'The Impact of Human Papilloma Virus (HPV) in Gynaecology', *Modern Phytotherapy - the Clinical Significance of Tea Tree and Other Essential Oils*, vol. 1 of the proceedings of a two day conference at Macquarie University, Sydney Dec. 1 & 2, 1990

Merry, K.A., 'Composition of Oils from *Melaleuca alternifolia, Melaleuca linariifolia, Melaleuca dissitisflora*. Implications for the Australian Standard, Oil of Melaleuca - Terpinen-4-ol Type', *Modern Phytotherapy - the Clinical Significance of Tea Tree and Other Essential Oils*, vol. 2 of the proceedings of a two day conference at Macquarie University, Sydney, Dec. 1 & 2, 1990

Olsen, C. W., *Australian Tea Tree Oil First Aid Handbook*, Kali Press, Pegosa Spring, Colorado, 1991

Olsen, C. W., *Australian Tea Tree Oil Guide: First Aid Kit in a Bottle*, Kali Press, Pagaso Springs, Colorado, 1997

Pena, Eduardo, 'Melaleuca Alternifolia Oil: It Use for Trichomonal Vaginitis and Other Vaginal Infections', *Journal of Obstetrics and Gynecology* 19 (1962), p. 792-95.

Penfold, Arthur and F. R. Morrison, 'Australian Tea Trees of Economic Value', *Technological Museum Bulletin*, vol. 14, 1929

Penfold, Author & F.R. Morrison, 'Some Notes of the Essential Oil of Melaleuca Alternifolia', *Australian Journal of Pharmacy*, March 1937, pp 274

Poucher, W.A., 'Tea Tree Oil', *Perfumes, Cosmetics and Soap*, 4th ed., 1:370, 1936

Puotinen, C. J., *Nature's Antiseptic: Tea Tree Oil and Grape Seed Extract*, Keats Publishing, New Canaan, Connecticut, 1997

Ryan, R., 'Oil of *Melaleuca alternifolia* Dissolved in Liquid Carbon Dioxide Propellant (Bactigas™) Used for the Control of Bacteria and Fungi in Air Conditioning Systems', *Modern Phytotherapy - the Clinical Significance of Tea Tree and Other Essential Oils*, vol. 2 of the proceedings of a two day conference at Macquarie University, Sydney, Dec. 1 & 2, 1990

Sachs, Prof. R., '*Melaleuca alternifolia*: An Estimate of its Potential as a Crop for California', *Modern Phytotherapy - the Clinical Significance of Tea Tree and Other Essential Oils*, vol. 2 of the proceedings of a two day conference at Macquarie University, Sydney, Dec. 1 & 2, 1990

Serrentino, Jo, *The Handbook of Essential Oils*, Literary Dimension, Quebec, Canada 1994

Serrentino, Jo, *How Natural Remedies Work*, Literary Dimension, Quebec, Canada 1990

Setright, R., 'A Phytotherapeutic Approach to the Immune System and Viral Infections', *Modern Phytotherapy - the Clinical Significance of Tea Tree and Other Essential Oils*, vol. 1 of the proceedings of a two day conference at Macquarie University, Sydney, Dec. 1 & 2, 1990

Shemesh, A. L. and W.L. Mayo, 'Tea Tree Oil - natural antiseptic and fungicide', *International Journal of Alternative and Complementary Medicine*, p.12, Dec. 1991

Stewart, D., 'The Scientific Basis and Clinical Significance of Essential Oil Use in Phytotherapy', *Modern Phytotherapy - the Clinical Significance of Tea Tree and Other Essential Oils*, vol. 1 of the proceedings of a two day conference at Macquarie University, Sydney, Dec. 1 & 2, 1990

Tisserand, M., *Aromatherapy for Women*. Thornsons, Ltd., Wellingborough, Northamptonshire, England, 1985.

Tisserand, Robert, *The Art of Aromatherapy*. Destiny Books, Rochester, Vermont, 1977.

Tisserand, Robert 'Athlete's Foot', *International Journal of Aromatherapy* 2.3, p. 19, 1989

Tyler, V.E., L.R. Brady, J.E. Robbers et al., *Pharmacognosy* (Eighth edition). Lea & Febiger, Philadelphia, 1981.

Walker, M., 'Clinical Investigation of Australian Melaleuca alternifolia for a Variety of Common Foot Problems', *Current Pediatry*, April 1972

Williams, Dr. L., 'The Modern Tea Tree Oil Story', *Modern Phytotherapy - the Clinical Significance of Tea Tree and Other Essential Oils*, vol. 1 of the proceedings of a two day conference at Macquarie University, Sydney, Dec. 1 & 2, 1990

Williams, Dr. L., 'Selection and Breeding of Superior Strains of Melaleuca Species to Produce Low Cost, High Quality Tea Tree Oil', *Modern Phytotherapy - the Clinical Significance of Tea Tree and Other Essential Oils*, vol. 2 of the proceedings of a two day conference at Macquarie University, Sydney, Dec. 1 & 2, 1990

Winters, Sir Jason, *Breakthrough: In Search of an Australian Legend, Miracle Healing Oil of the Ages*, Vinton Publishing, Las Vegas, Nevada, 1986

Woodword, Valerie Ann, *The Fragrant Pharmacy: a complete guide to aromatherapy and essential oils*, Bantam, London, England, 1991

Index

To Write to the Authors

If you wish to write the authors, please write in care of AGES Publications™ and we will forward your request. Both the authors and publisher appreciate hearing from you and learning of the benefits and enjoyment you received from this book. AGES Publications™ cannot guarantee that every letter written can be answered by the authors, but all will be forwarded.
Please write to:

In the U.S. write to: Ken Vegotsky
c/o AGES Publications™
1623 Military Road, #203-TT,
Niagara Falls, NY 14304-1745

Please enclose a self-addressed, stamped envelop for reply, and $3.00 to cover costs.

In Canada write to: Ken Vegotsky
AGES Publications™
1054-2 Centre St., #153-TT,
Thornhill, Ontario, L4J 8E5.
Canada

Please enclose a self-addressed, stamped envelope for reply, and $4.00 to cover costs.

If outside the U.S.A. or Canada, enclose international postal reply coupon with a self-addressed envelope and $3.00 U.S. to cover costs.

About the author's...

Dr. Elvis Ali, B.Sc., N.D., Dipl. Ac., M.R.N.

...is a licensed Naturopathic Doctor and a Registered Nutritional Consultant, R.N.C. He graduated with a B.Sc. in Biology, in 1979 and became one of Canada's first full time registered undergraduates in the field of Naturopathic Medicine. He received a Doctorate in Naturopathic Medicine in 1987 from the Canadian College of Naturopathic Medicine, one of only five accredited schools offering a four year full time program in Naturopathic Medicine in the U.S.A. and Canada. Elvis has been in private practice for over 12 years specializing in Chinese Medicine, Nutrition and Sports Medicine.

"My mission is to educate the public and be a spokesperson for complementary health and wellness options and continued research in the field of herbal remedies, bringing safe and non-intrusive options into the public domain," says Dr. Ali.

He has written numerous articles on nutrition, stress and alternative healing options.

One of North America's premier natural remedy and supplement companies, Swiss Herbal Remedies, retains Dr. Ali as their resident Naturopath with ongoing responsibility for product research and development. He is currently making presentations in the U.S.A. and Canada, in addition to numerous media appearances on radio and TV, as his commitment to increase the health and wellness of every man, woman and child in the U.S.A. and Canada.

He is married and the father of two children.

To arrange a keynote, seminar and/or workshop presentation by Dr. Ali, call the contact coordinator at (519) 396-9553.

About the author's...

Dr. George F. Grant, M.Sc., M.Ed., Ed.D., C. Chem., C.I.H.

...is a multi-talented scientist who pioneered the research on Beta Endorphins, anticancer drugs, Lactobacilus viridescens model system to investigate microbial greening, HPLC analysis of B vitamins, GC-MS drug identification of potential drugs for prostate cancer, indoor air quality problems as related to Tight Building Syndrome and his well known research on Stress Management and Wellness.
He is listed in the International Who's Who of Professional's. Dr.Grant holds two patents on Modified Atmosphere Packaging (MAP) and Liposomal Weight Management spray.

He is the author of several published research articles, book reviews, conference presentations, and hundreds of public speaking engagements across North America.

Dr. Grant is an active member of five professional organizations in the U.S.A. and Canada. He is a licensed Analytical Chemist, Certified Industrial Hygienist, Food/Nutrition Scientist, College Professor and Consultant for several international firms.

He is married and a father of two boys.

Dr. Grant is known nationally and internationally as a wellness coach. He does presentations in Seattle, Washington and Toronto, Ontario, Canada.

For speaking engagements, call (905) 737-1788.

About the
author's...

Dr. Selim Nakla, M.D.

...is a medical graduate from the oldest university in the world, Alexandria University, Egypt. He has been published in the American Journal of Obstetrics, Gynecology and Neunatology. For the past eleven years he has been practicing a blend of traditional and holistic medicine for health management in his practice. His primary focus includes physiotherapy, rehabilitation medicine, acupuncture and alternative medicine.

Dr. Nakla's presentations currently focus on nutrition and alternative medicine. His primary focus is helping people help themselves, using as non-intrusive a style as possible, for their health and well-being. He has presented in the U.S.A., Canada, Italy and Egypt.

Don Patel, B.Sc., M.R.T., C.N.M.T.

...is a certified Nuclear Medicine technologist in the U.S.A. and Canada. He has 25 years of experience in the diagnostic field of Nuclear Medicine, including Nuclear Cardiology.

He is currently investigating wellness products and alternative methods which can be helpful in prevention of cardiac disease and enhance general health and well-being for the adult population.

About the author's...

Ken Vegotsky, B.Sc.

...is a professional speaker, author and entrepreneur who has given keynote addresses and seminars in the U.S.A. and Canada. He has been featured in print, radio and TV in the U.S.A., Canada, Australia, New Zealand, United Kingdom and a host of other countries.

"Ken is the Victor Frankl of our day," noted Dottie Walters, President Walters Speakers Bureau International and author of Speak & Grow Rich.

Mark Victor Hansen, New York Times #1 bestselling co-author of the Chicken Soup for the Soul Series, says Ken's work is, **"Brilliant and illuminating."**

"In recognition of being seen as a model of courage and hope for others, who demonstrates to all of us the nobility of the human spirit," begins the Clarke Foundation nomination of Ken for a *Courage to Come Back Award*. These awards were originated by the St. Francis Health Foundation of Pittsburgh, Pennsylvania.

Ken has served on the boards of NACPAC (affiliate of the American Chronic Pain Association), a community information service and a half–way home for mentally challenged people in transition. After numerous inspirational speeches, Vegotsky was encouraged by listeners to tell his story.

In his National Bestseller, *The Ultimate Power,* Ken shares his captivating first-person account of his near-death experience, garnished with proven keys for unlocking your personal power. Discover *How to Make Love With Life!*™ and you'll feel embraced by caring and compassion as you share his moving experience.

To arrange a keynote, seminar and/or workshop presentation by Ken Vegotsky, call the contact coordinator at (519) 396-9553.

Coming Soon

Stress Free Living

222 Ways to Live Stress Free

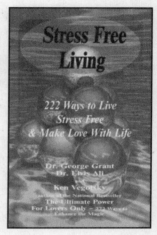

ISBN 1-886508-04-6

$7.95 for this Gift Card Book

Discover...

Powerful ways to reduce stress and
enrich your life

Magical ways to quickly bust stress

How to access your **Mind–Body–Soul** connection to
relieve stress

Nourishing insights to nurture your soul and
help you live fully in the moment

Natural healing and alternative therapies to live stress free
and enhance your life today

An Entertaining & Fun Way to
Discover 222 Ways to Live Stress Free

Dr. Elvis Ali, Dr. George Grant
Dr. Selim Nakla
Don Patel & Ken Vegotsky
Those who brought you The Tea Tree Oil Bible

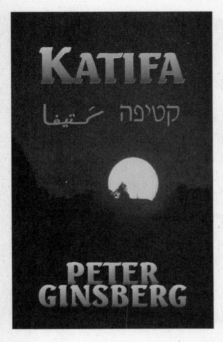

When retired operative John Quick died, he left his housekeeper Emma Gwynn his estate, his past and a sniper's rifle to kill the man who murdered him. Suddenly thrust into a wilderness of mirrors no less treacherous with the ending of the cold war, Emma Gwynn descends into a twilight world of deception fraught with the ghosts of combatants long since dead, but clearly unaware of their passing.

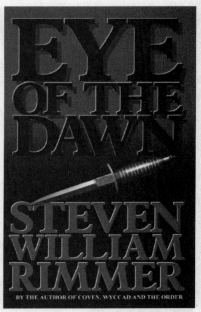

EYE
OF THE
DAWN

ISBN 1-886508-09-7

$6.99

Fiction/Mystery

by Steven William Rimmer

Author of Coven • Wyccad • The Order

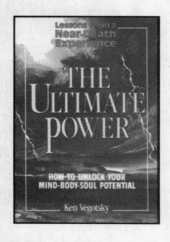

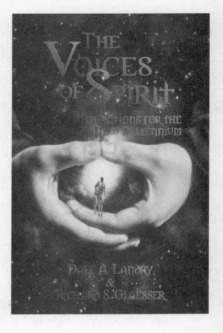

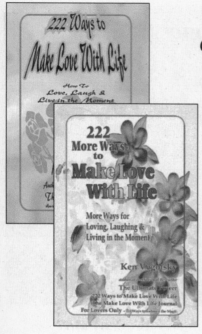

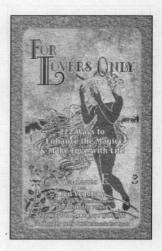

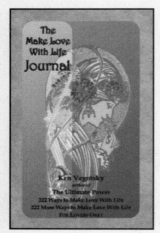

Order Form

	Qty	Price	Total
The Make Love With Life Journal over 100 inspirational & motivational sayings		$7.95	
222 Ways to Make Love With Life How To Love, Laugh and Live in the Moment		$7.95	
222 More Ways to Make Love With Life More Ways for Loving… Living in the Moment		$7.95	
For Lovers Only 222 Ways to Enhance the Magic		$7.95	
Stress Free Living – 222 Ways to Live Stress Free		$7.95	
The Ultimate Power How to Unlock Your Mind Body Soul Potential		$14.95	
The Voices of Spirit Predictions for the New Millennium		$12.95	
Katifa speculative fiction		$6.95	
Eye of the Dawn fiction/mystery		$6.99	
The Tea Tree Oil Bible Your Essential Guide		$7.95	
Hypnotic Journey of Gentle Surrender Relaxation techniques – Audio Tape		$9.95	
($3.00 for 1st + $0.50 for each additional item) Shipping			
Total			

Name_____

Address _____

City _____ZIP _____

Phone _____

Please make certified check/money order payable to and send to
Adi, Gaia, Esalen Publications Inc.
1623 Military Rd. #203-TT, Niagara Falls, NY 14304-1745

VISA ☐   MasterCard ☐   American Express ☐

Card #: _____Exp. Date: _____

Signature: _____

North America – Order Toll Free 1 800 263-1991
Trade and Bulk order enquiries welcomed

Order Form

	Qty	Price	Total
The Make Love With Life Journal over 100 inspirational & motivational sayings		$7.95	
222 Ways to Make Love With Life How To Love, Laugh and Live in the Moment		$7.95	
222 More Ways to Make Love With Life More Ways for Loving… Living in the Moment		$7.95	
For Lovers Only 222 Ways to Enhance the Magic		$7.95	
Stress Free Living – 222 Ways to Live Stress Free		$7.95	
The Ultimate Power How to Unlock Your Mind Body Soul Potential		$14.95	
The Voices of Spirit Predictions for the New Millennium		$12.95	
Katifa speculative fiction		$6.95	
Eye of the Dawn fiction/mystery		$6.99	
The Tea Tree Oil Bible Your Essential Guide		$7.95	
Hypnotic Journey of Gentle Surrender Relaxation techniques – Audio Tape		$9.95	
($3.00 for 1st + $0.50 for each additional item) **Shipping**			
		Total	

Name_____

Address _____

City _____ZIP _____

Phone _____

Please make certified check/money order payable to and send to
Adi, Gaia, Esalen Publications Inc.
1623 Military Rd. #203-TT, Niagara Falls, NY 14304-1745

VISA ☐   MasterCard ☐   American Express ☐

Card #: _____Exp. Date: _____

Signature: _____

North America – Order Toll Free 1 800 263-1991
Trade and Bulk order enquiries welcomed